6

Weeks to
Get Out the
FAT

Also by the
AMERICAN HEART ASSOCIATION

American Heart Association Cookbook, 5th Edition

American Heart Association Low-Fat, Low-Cholesterol Cookbook

American Heart Association Low-Salt Cookbook

American Heart Association Quick and Easy Cookbook

American Heart Association Kids' Cookbook

American Heart Association Brand Name Fat and Cholesterol Counter

American Heart Association Family Guide to Stroke

With the American Cancer Society Living Well, Staying Well

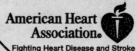

American Heart
Association.

Fighting Heart Disease and Stroke

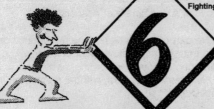

Weeks to Get Out the FAT

An Easy-to-Follow Program for Trimming the Fat from Your Diet

Clarkson Potter/Publishers
New York

Your contribution to the American Heart Association supports research that helps make publications like this possible. For more information call 1-800-AHA-USA1 (1-800-242-8721).

Published by Clarkson Potter/Publishers
Member of the Crown Publishing Group.

Random House, Inc. New York, Toronto, London, Sydney, Auckland
www.randomhouse.com

CLARKSON N. POTTER is a trademark and POTTER and colophon are registered trademarks of Random House, Inc.

Originally published by Times Books in 1996

Printed in the United States of America

Book design, page makeup, and text composition by Leon Bolognese & Associates, Inc.

Library of Congress Cataloging-in-Publication Data
American Heart Association 6 weeks to get out the fat: an easy-to-follow program for trimming the fat from your diet / American Heart Association.—1st ed.
　　1. Low-fat diet. I. Title: 6 weeks to get out the fat
RM237.7.A445　　 1996
613.2'8—dc20　　 96-12855

ISBN 0-8129-2747-8

10　9　8

ACKNOWLEDGMENTS

Food is an important part of a balanced diet.

—Fran Lebowitz

Writing this book was just plain fun. We laughed, we wrote, we ate. In the process, each of us learned at least a dozen new ways to cut down on fat. We learned how easy it is to make lots of small changes in our eating that add up to big savings in cholesterol. And we learned The Big News—that *all* foods (even our high-fat favorites) fit into a heart-healthy diet.

This book is our bag of tricks. It's just about everything we could think of to help you eat with your heart in mind. It comes with our hopes that these tips will be beneficial in your quest for a full and healthy life, free of heart disease and stroke.

First to receive applause and our eternal thanks are Ruth Ann Carpenter, M.S., R.D., and Sara Kelling, M.P.H., R.D., the nutrition experts who researched or devised the hundreds of fat-busting tips in this book. For Ruth Ann and Sara, eating for a healthy heart is second nature—they're staff members of the Cooper Institute for Aerobics Research, a nonprofit preventive medicine research and education center in Dallas, Texas.

American Heart Association Senior Editor Jane Anneken Ruehl deserves at least two curtain calls. She assembled the team of experts, writers, and editors, then managed the development process from concept to completed book. An armload of roses goes to Editor Janice Roth Moss, who painstakingly copyedited every word. And kudos to writer Pat Naegele, who polished the words of the experts to a high gloss.

Mary Winston, R.D., Ph.D., AHA Senior Science Consultant, deserves to take a deep bow. She checked and double-checked the scientific accuracy of every fat-cutting tip in this book.

We hope you enjoy reading this book as much as we enjoyed putting it together. *Bon appétit!*

CONTENTS

INTRODUCTION

We wrote 6 Weeks to Get Out the Fat to help you cut the fat and cholesterol in your diet. When you opened this book, you joined millions of other Americans who want and need to reduce their risk of heart attack by lowering their blood cholesterol level. How do they do that? By cutting down on the total fat, saturated fat, and cholesterol in their diet.

As you'll see on these pages, "getting out the fat" is easier than you might think. In fact, you'll find hundreds of simple ways to trim total fat, saturated fat, and cholesterol. We tried to make this book easy to use, practical to apply, and flexible—we want it to fit in with any lifestyle. Of course, every idea won't help every person. However, you'll find plenty of suggestions that definitely will be helpful to you. It's simply a matter of trial and error. So whether you just want to fine-tune your eating plan or give it a complete overhaul, 6 Weeks to Get Out the Fat can work for you!

♡ High Fat, High Risk

Everyone knows that eating too much fat (especially saturated fat) and cholesterol is not good for your health. First, because fat is so concentrated in calories, it can lead to obesity when you eat too much of it. Being obese can in turn increase your blood cholesterol, your blood pressure, and your risk of diabetes. Both saturated fat and dietary cholesterol boost your blood cholesterol. Saturated fat is the big culprit. Foods from animal sources contain both saturated fat and cholesterol. So, when you cut back one, you often cut back the other. High blood cholesterol is a major risk factor for heart attack and stroke. Other risk factors include high blood pressure, smoking, and physical inactivity.

It's clear, then, that you can help your heart as well as your general health by cutting down on fat in your diet. (You'll also trim your waistline.) The truth is that the average American gets 33% of his or her daily calories from fat. At the American Heart Association, we recommend getting less than 30% of your calories from fat. And we're not alone. Many health experts support this recommendation. Although you want to keep fat intake low, you don't want to cut *all* the fat from your diet. Everyone should have a *little* fat for good health. What you really need is a balanced diet made up of a wide variety of foods.

♡ Pyramid Power

The American Heart Association's Healthy Heart Food Pyramid is a guide to help you eat the right amounts of a variety of foods from the different food groups. It can help you choose foods that provide all the nutrients you need without too much fat, saturated fat, and cholesterol. You can see immedi-

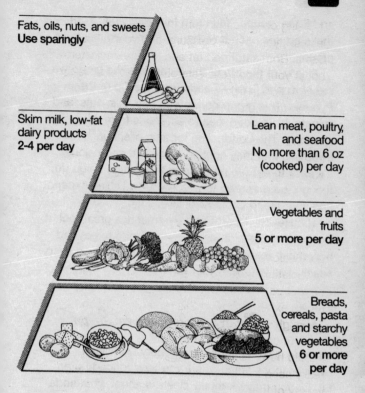

Fats, oils, nuts, and sweets
Use sparingly

Skim milk, low-fat
dairy products
2-4 per day

Lean meat, poultry,
and seafood
**No more than 6 oz
(cooked) per day**

Vegetables and
fruits
5 or more per day

Breads,
cereals, pasta
and starchy
vegetables
**6 or more
per day**

ately that the Breads, Cereals, Pasta, and Starchy
Vegetables group and the Vegetables and Fruits
group make up the large majority of the Pyramid.
Why? Because foods in these groups are generally
low in fat and high in nutrition. For that reason, most
of your diet should consist of foods from these two
groups. In fact, these groups form the foundation of
any heart-healthy eating plan.

On the next level are the Skim Milk and Low-Fat
Dairy Products and the Lean Meat, Poultry, Seafood,

and Eggs groups. You need fewer servings from these groups each day than from the two major groups.

Finally, at the top of the Pyramid is the group we call Now and Then—Foods from the Tip of the Pyramid. This group consists of fats, oils, nuts, and sweets. It's a good idea to eat foods from this group sparingly. The bottom line for fats, oils, nuts, and sweets is that they contain mostly fat and calories. It's easy to eat too much from this group. If you do, though, be prepared to watch your waistline expand and your blood cholesterol level soar.

The Healthy Heart Food Pyramid is a great tool. It can help you decide what kind of foods to eat and how much to eat. Every meal is a choice. So is every snack. You vote with your fork.

♡ Fat-Busting: Where to Start?

You may already know your dietary "Achilles' heels"—those areas where you tend to load up on fat. Or you may be totally clueless about what adds those pounds around the middle and raises that blood cholesterol level.

In the following chapter, we'll show you how to assess your current food choices. We'll also help you identify ways to lower your intake of total fat, saturated fat, and cholesterol. You'll find several tools to help you use this book to the max. For example, you'll learn how to track your food intake so you'll know your fat and cholesterol problem areas. The "Fat IQ" quiz, starting on page 12, can help you spot areas where you tend to overdo it in the fat department. With this knowledge, you can zero in on your biggest one or two problem areas. Just remember to take it easy. You don't want the changes you're making to vaporize after just a few weeks. Instead, you want them to last a lifetime.

♡ À la Carte

The main part of this book is six "do-it-yourself" fat-busting chapters. Each chapter is designed for one week and deals with a different aspect of reducing fat. Week 1 gets you off to a quick start with easy changes you can make to pack a big fat-reduction punch. In Week 2 you'll learn how much of each type of food to eat. Week 3 offers guidelines on putting together well-balanced, low-fat meals. Week 4 has scads of heart-healthy cooking tips. In Week 5, you'll learn how to budget your fat intake. And, finally, Week 6 is your fat-cutting wrap-up, with last-minute tips and tests to see if you "got it." Get it?

We arranged the information in each chapter according to the food groups found in the Healthy Heart Food Pyramid, plus a section called Eating Out—Eating Healthy. We've included information on shopping, cooking, and eating with your heart in mind. And each chapter is packed with fat-fighting strategies you can start right away.

How you use this book is up to you. Feel free to mix and match or even skip around. For example, you may want to zero in on a single food group, say the one that includes milk and dairy products. If so, just find the section on the Skim Milk and Low-Fat Dairy Products group in each chapter. Work on a few tips for that food group in Week 1. After you've mastered those, go on to Week 2, and so on.

On the other hand, you may want to read each chapter from start to finish before choosing a few suggestions to work on. Whichever method you choose is fine. But no matter how you read the book, the only way you'll succeed in cutting the fat in your diet is to actually *make the changes*. Reading, by itself, will *not* lower your fat intake or your blood cholesterol level!

♡ *Just Desserts*

Even though this book is titled *6 Weeks to Get Out the Fat*, you can take longer than a week per chapter if you need to. On the other hand, you may breeze through a chapter in less than a week. That's especially likely if you're concentrating on making changes in only one food group. But if you move through the book too quickly, your heart-helping changes may not last. If you go too slowly, you could get bored and kiss off the changes altogether. There's no "magic" in the six-week time frame. The magic is in you and your determination. Give it a try. You'll find the rewards are sweet.

Taking Stock: How Much Fat, Saturated Fat, and Cholesterol Are You Eating?

et's face it: Fat tastes good. It's part of what makes you feel full and satisfied after a meal. Your body needs some fat to function properly. But it needs only a very small amount.

When you pull up to a service station to buy gasoline, the pump shows how much fuel you're putting into your car's gas tank. In fact, it shuts off automatically when the tank is full. Unfortunately, your body doesn't have an automatic shutoff valve to tell you when you've eaten enough fat for the day. So it's easy to "overfill" your fat tank.

In this chapter, we've given you three tools—a food diary, a fat-intake questionnaire, and a quiz to find out how balanced your diet is. These will help you determine how much fat, saturated fat, and cholesterol you eat every day. Armed with the knowledge you gain from each of these, you can use the rest of the book to find out how to trim the fat and cut the cholesterol—for life.

♡ Are You Eating High on the Hog?

Keeping a food diary is a great way to see what you really are eating each day. Take a look at the Sample Food Diary on pages 4 and 5. Then turn to pages 6 and 7 for your own diary form. It's designed to help you track your daily fat, cholesterol, and calorie intake. What you learn may surprise you.

A food diary is a really helpful tool. Besides letting you track the total amount of fat, saturated fat, and cholesterol you eat every day, it also helps you identify which foods and food groups are full of those substances. For example, you might have eaten a doughnut for breakfast, thinking you were avoiding the fat and cholesterol of a fried egg. But did you realize that an average glazed doughnut has nearly 13 grams of fat? That's more than many low-fat dinner entrées!

♡ How to Keep a Food Diary

Using a food diary takes a little practice. As with any other new tool, you need to learn the tricks that will help you be successful. Here are some ideas to get you started.

❑ Make a few photocopies of the blank diary pages. Record what you eat for several *typical* weekdays and at least one weekend day. That may help you identify when you are likely to eat more—Sunday brunch maybe?

❑ List every morsel that goes into your mouth. Start with the first thing you eat in the morning and list everything—including snacks—until the time you go to sleep.

❑ Describe *in detail* everything you eat and drink. Don't forget such items as the mayonnaise on sandwiches and the dressings on salads. If you taste as you cook, be sure to include all those extra spoonfuls, too.

❑ Write down each food and beverage *immediately* after you eat or drink it. If you wait until the end of the day, you'll forget some of the details. Just carry a copy of the daily diary pages in your pocket or purse.

❑ Write down the amount you ate or drank. Try to be accurate about your portion sizes.

❑ Fill in as many of the remaining blanks as you can. Read food labels and check easy-to-use guides to find the fat, saturated fat, cholesterol, and calorie amounts for each food you eat. One guide is the American Heart Association's *Brand Name Fat and Cholesterol Counter*.

❑ Add up your totals for the day.

❑ Compare those numbers with the ones listed on the "Fat Grams by Calorie Levels" chart on page 8 as recommended for your caloric intake.

If your numbers are lower than those listed, you're already on the road to a heart-healthy diet. Even so, you'll find that this book is filled with great ideas to help you cut your fat intake even further. If your totals are higher than those numbers, this book can

Sample Food Diary

Food Description	Amount Eaten	Total Fat (g)*	Saturated Fat (g)*	Cholesterol (mg)†	Calories
Breakfast (at home; in a rush)					
Frosted flake cereal	1½ cups	0.1	0.0	0.0	220
Milk, 2%	½ cup	2.3	1.5	9.0	60
Orange juice	1 cup	0.1	0.0	0.0	112
Coffee	1 cup	0.0	0.0	0.0	0.0
Half & half cream	1 tbsp	1.7	1.1	6.0	20
Morning Snack (in office)					
Glazed cake doughnut	1 medium	12.6	2.9	17.0	244
Decaf coffee	1 cup	0.0	0.0	0.0	0.0
Powdered coffee creamer	2 tsp	1.4	1.4	0.0	22
Lunch (brought from home)					
Ham and cheese sandwich					
Wheat bread	2 slices	2.0	0.0	0.0	122
Ham, lean	2 oz	2.3	0.8	3.0	119
Swiss cheese	2 slices	14.2	5.8	30.0	190
Mayo (regular, I think)	1 tbsp	11.0	1.6	8.0	99
Mustard	2 tsp	0.4	0.0	0.0	8
Potato chips	1½-oz bag	14.7	4.7	0.0	228
Apple	1 medium	0.5	0.1	0.0	81
Cola drink	12-oz can	0.0	0.0	0.0	151

Food Description	Amount Eaten	Total Fat (g)*	Satura-ted Fat (g)*	Choles-terol (mg)†	Calories
Afternoon Snack (from vending machine)					
Milk chocolate bar	1½ oz	13.5	8.1	10.0	226
Dinner (on the way home from day care)					
Fast-food quarter-pound burger w/cheese	1	20.7	8.1	86	410
Diet cola	large	0.0	0.0	0.0	0.0
French fries (finished my son's order)	¼ regular order	3.0	1.3	2.0	55
Ketchup	2 tsp	0.0	0.0	0.0	12
Evening Snacks (at home)					
Jelly beans	10 pieces	0.1	0.0	0.0	104
Low-fat frozen yogurt, vanilla	½ cup	4.0	2.5	2.0	114
Chocolate syrup	1 tbsp	0.2	0.1	0.0	41
	TOTAL	104.8	40	200	2,638

*grams
†milligrams

Food Diary

Date	Food Description	Amount Eaten	

	Total Fat (g)	Saturated Fat (g)	Cholesterol (mg)	Calories
TOTAL				

Fat Grams by Calorie Levels

Calorie Level	Maximum Total Fat Grams (30% of calories)	Saturated Fat (10% of calories)	Saturated Fat (7% of calories)
1,200	40	13	9
1,500	50	17	12
1,800	60	20	14
2,000	67	22	16
2,200	73	24	17
2,500	83	28	19
3,000	100	33	23

really help you. Look at the foods listed in your diary and circle the ones that contribute the most fat. Then read this book with those items in mind. You'll find dozens of ways to trim the fat from most of the foods you like. That way, you can keep enjoying them—but without risking your good health.

♡ Labels Make Good Reading

If you eat packaged foods, figuring the fat, saturated fat, and cholesterol is easy. Simply read the nutrient information on the package. Look at the sample label on page 9. You'll see that total fat, saturated fat, dietary cholesterol, and sodium are all clearly listed.

WARNING: Be sure to check portion sizes. The amount you eat may not always match what the

Nutrition Facts

Serving Size 1/2 cup (114g)
Servings Per Container 4

Amount Per Serving

Calories 90   Calories from Fat 30

	% Daily Value*
Total Fat 3g	**5%**
Saturated Fat 0g	**0%**
Cholesterol 0mg	**0%**
Sodium 300g	**13%**
Total Carbohydrate 13mg	**4%**
Dietary Fiber 3g	**12%**
Sugars 3g	
Protein 3g	

Vitamin A	80%	• Vitamin C	60%
Calcium	4%	• Iron	4%

*Percent Daily Values are based on 2,000 calorie diet. Your daily values may be higher or lower depending on your calorie needs:

		Calories	2,000	2,500
Total Fat	Less than		65g	80g
Sat Fat	Less than		20g	25mg
Cholesterol	Less than		300mg	300mg
Sodium	Less than		2,400mg	2,400mg
Total Carbohydrate			300g	375g
Fiber			25g	30g

Calories per gram:

Fat 9   •   Carbohydrate 4   •   Protein 4

food label lists as a normal serving. For example, a food label may say one serving is two cookies, but you may normally eat four. In that case, you'll need to double the amounts given for calories, total fat, saturated fat, and cholesterol when you log your entry.

♡ Diary Dilemma

Many people enjoy keeping a daily diary—whether it's what they did on vacation or what they ate for an entire week. Others, however, just don't like to write things down. A food diary is just one tool to help you be aware of what you're eating. We encourage you to keep a food diary so you can look closely at your own food intake. If, however, you don't want to complete the diary, that's okay. You can still use this book. Just go on to the next section and take a look at "Your Fat IQ."

♡ Your Fat IQ (Intake Quotient)

On the following pages, you'll find a self-scoring quiz designed to help you discover your *usual* total fat, saturated fat, and cholesterol intake. It's not like the food diary—it won't tell you how many grams of fat and milligrams of cholesterol you usually eat. It's a general guide to help you find areas where you can make changes to help reduce the fat, saturated fat, and cholesterol in your diet. It can also point you to parts of this book that may be of special interest to you.

The quiz covers each of the six categories of food we talk about in this book. For each category, five specific questions about your food-related habits are listed in the left column. Answer each question by choosing one of the responses given. Then write the corresponding number of points in the space provided. When you have answered all the questions about a food category, add your scores to get your total for that category. Then add all your totals (see page 24) to get your grand total. The numbers themselves are arbitrary. A 20, for example, is not twice as "good" as a 10. The cutoff points for the total score are also arbitrary. There is no magic in the number 60, for example. A score of 61 is not far removed from the "30 to 60" category. The quiz is not a "scientific instrument." It's just one way to help you get an idea of the sources of fat and cholesterol in your diet. It is also a road map to guide you through the book.

As you take this quiz, consider the following:

◆ If you don't eat every food listed in an entry, score yourself for the ones you do eat.

◆ Try to complete this questionnaire at home. You may need to check a few food labels in your pantry and refrigerator to be able to answer some of these questions.

Again, we urge you to complete this quiz. If, however, you want to jump right into the program, just turn to page 34 and begin with Week 1. For everyone else, get your pencils ready. Let's begin.

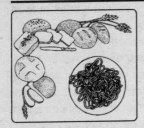

Breads, Cereals, Pasta, and Starchy Vegetables

How often do you . . .	1 point
Eat ready-to-eat cereals with more than 3 grams of fat per serving?	Often
Eat quick breads, biscuits, muffins, waffles, pancakes, corn bread, etc.?	Often
Add margarine, oil, or butter when cooking or eating pasta, rice, cereal, noodles, waffles, pancakes, etc.?	Always or usually
Add margarine, butter, cheese, and/or sour cream to starchy vegetables (potatoes, corn, lima beans, etc.)?	Always or usually
Eat starchy beans or peas (lentils; kidney, lima, garbanzo, or pinto beans; split peas) without added fat?	Rarely or never

3 points	5 points	Score
Occasionally	Rarely or never	
		_____
Occasionally	Rarely or never	
		_____
Occasionally	Rarely or never	
		_____
Occasionally	Rarely or never	
		_____
Occasionally (several times per month)	Often (at least once a week)	
		_____
	Total Score	_____

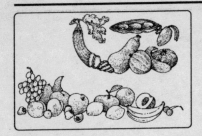

Vegetables and Fruits *

How often do you ...	1 point
Eat marinated vegetables or vegetable salads made with regular dressing?	Often
Eat high-fat dips or spreads (peanut butter, sour cream, cream cheese, etc.) with vegetables or fruit?	Often
Add margarine, butter, or cheese when cooking or eating vegetables?	Usually or always
Eat vegetables in a cream sauce?	Often
Eat fried or sautéed vegetables?	Often

* Starchy vegetables, such as corn, potatoes, and dried beans, are incuded in the Breads, Cereals, Pasta, and Starchy Vegetables group (see pages 12 and 13).

3 points	5 points	Score
Occasionally	Rarely or never	
		————
Occasionally	Rarely or never	
		————
Occasionally	Rarely or never	
		————
Occasionally	Rarely or never	————
Occasionally	Rarely or never	————
	Total Score	————

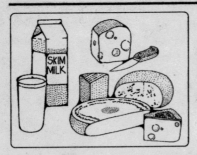

*Skim Milk and
Low-Fat
Dairy Products*

How often do you . . .	1 point
Drink whole or 2% milk?	Often, or never drink any type of milk
Eat yogurt (frozen or refrigerated) made with whole milk?	Often
Eat regular hard or processed cheeses?	Often
Eat regular soft cheeses (cottage cheese, ricotta, cream cheese, etc.)?	Often
Use regular sour cream, cream, or half-and-half?	Often

3 points	5 points	Score
Occasionally	Rarely or never	_____
Occasionally	Rarely or never	_____
Occasionally	Rarely or never	_____
Occasionally	Rarely or never	_____
Occasionally	Rarely or never	_____
	Total Score	_____

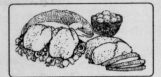

Lean Meat, Poultry, Seafood, and Eggs

Do you . . .	1 point
Eat beef, pork, lamb, or veal?*	Usually choose Prime cuts, regular hamburger, brisket, ribs, etc.
Eat turkey or chicken?*	Usually choose fried poultry, poultry cooked with skin and skin eaten, or regular ground poultry.
Usually cook meat, poultry, or seafood by . . .?*	Frying.
Eat breakfast meats or cold cuts?*	Usually choose regular sausage, bacon, regular hot dogs, bologna, salami, liverwurst, etc.
Usually eat eggs?	7 or more egg yolks per week.

*Give yourself a score of 5 if you eat meat or poultry fewer than four times per month.

3 points	5 points	Score
Usually choose lean or extra-lean cuts or lean ground meats.	Always choose lean or extra-lean cuts or lean ground meats.	_____
Usually choose baked, broiled, or grilled poultry; poultry cooked with skin and skin eaten; or lean ground poultry.	Always choose baked, broiled, or grilled poultry; poultry cooked without skin and skin not eaten; or lean ground poultry.	_____
Baking, grilling, or broiling. Meat is untrimmed; poultry is cooked with skin.	Baking, grilling, or broiling. Meat is trimmed of fat; poultry is skinned before cooking.	_____
Usually choose Canadian bacon, lean roast beef or ham, turkey breast, or reduced-fat cold cuts or hot dogs.	Always choose Canadian bacon, lean roast beef or ham, turkey breast, or reduced-fat cold cuts or hot dogs.	_____
4 to 6 egg yolks per week.	Fewer than 4 egg yolks per week or use only egg whites or egg substitute.	_____
	Total Score	_____

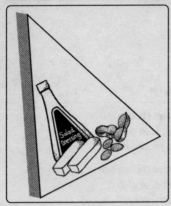

Now and Then—
Foods from
the Tip of the
Pyramid

How often do you . . .	1 point
Use butter or stick margarine for spreading?	Usually or always
Use lard, butter, or shortening for cooking?	Usually or always
Use regular dressings or regular mayonnaise?	Usually or always
Use regular coffee creamers?	Usually or always
Eat regular snack crackers, chips, nuts, cookies, cakes, pies, candies, or ice cream?	Often

3 points	5 points	Score
Occasionally	Rarely or never	_____
Occasionally	Rarely or never	_____
Occasionally	Rarely or never	_____
Occasionally	Rarely or never	_____
Occasionally	Rarely or never	
		_____
	Total Score	_____

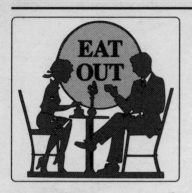

Eating Out—
Eating Healthy

How often do you . . .	1 point
Eat out each week?	Usually or always (more than three times a week)
Choose restaurants that offer low-fat items?	Rarely or never
Select grilled, baked, broiled, poached, or steamed entrées?	Rarely or never
Order salad dressing, creamy sauces, sour cream, or guacamole on the side?	Rarely or never
Feel confident that you make heart-healthy choices when eating out?	Rarely or never

3 points	5 points	Score
Occasionally (about three times a week)	Rarely or never (fewer than three times a week)	_____
Occasionally	Usually or always	_____
Occasionally	Usually or always	_____
Occasionally	Usually or always	_____
		_____
Occasionally	Usually or always	_____
		_____
	Total Score	_____

♡ Scoring Your Self-Test

In the space below, write your score for each of the six food categories.

My Score

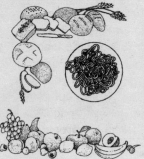

Breads, Cereals,
Pasta, and
Starchy Vegetables _____

Vegetables and
Fruits _____

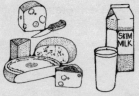

Skim Milk and
Low-Fat Dairy
Products _____

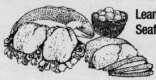

Lean Meat, Poultry,
Seafood, and Eggs _____

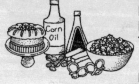

Now and Then—
Foods from the
Tip of the Pyramid _____

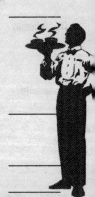

Eating Out—
Eating Healthy _____

GRAND TOTAL _____

If your grand total score is

30–60   You're eating your heart out! This score
means your diet is extremely high in fat,
saturated fat, and cholesterol. That could
lead to cardiovascular problems down the
line. Luckily, you can change your food
choices to create a more healthful eating
pattern. Start making changes in your diet
today. Begin by reviewing the chapter enti-
tled "Week 1: An Easy Takeoff" (page 34).
It contains lots of excellent hints for cutting
your fat intake quickly and easily. Don't try
to do everything at once. Just pick the tips
that fit your eating patterns and prefer-
ences. But remember, the more of these
changes you make, the more fat you can
cut from your diet. Take a couple of weeks
to work through this chapter, then gradually
do the same with the next five chapters.
Your good health may depend on it.

61–90   You need to reduce the fat, saturated fat,
and cholesterol in your diet. In fact, you
probably scored below 10 in several of the
food categories listed. To make improve-
ments, decide which category to work on
first and make gradual changes in just that
category. You can pick the area that needs
the most improvement or tackle the category that would be easiest to make
changes in. Begin with the suggestions in
your chosen category for Week 1. Then
progress at a comfortable pace to Week 6.

If necessary, you can spend more than one week working on a chapter. When you have knocked the fat out of the foods in one group, find another group that you want to work on and repeat the process. Your heart will love you for it!

91–120   You're already making some healthful eating choices—that's great news for your heart! To improve your diet even more, find the items on which you scored 1 or 3. Select several to modify, then take a look at the next six chapters. Simply find the food groups (for example, Skim Milk and Low-Fat Dairy Products and Eating Out—Eating Healthy) that contain your problem foods or habits. Starting with Week 1, look for specific fat-busting ideas in those categories. The rest of the material in each chapter offers other heart-healthy eating ideas.

121–150 Congratulations! You're already well on your way to a diet that is low in fat, saturated fat, and cholesterol. This book can help you fine-tune your eating plan even more. In *6 Weeks to Get Out the Fat,* you'll find a source that's chock-full of helpful tips and suggestions. The material in the chapters for Weeks 4 through 6 may be especially helpful to you. Browse through the following pages to find new ways to keep your fat and cholesterol intake in the help-your-heart range.

♡ A Healthy Diet Is a Balancing Act

Now that you're ready to take steps to reduce the fat, saturated fat, and cholesterol in what you eat, it's important to remember that fat-busting is not the whole ball game. You must also make sure you're getting all the nutrients your body needs for good health.

As an example, you might try to reduce the fat in your diet by eating only fruit and bread. True, your diet would certainly be low in fat. But that doesn't mean the diet would be good for you. While you cut your fat, you must also make sure you're eating a balanced diet. That means eating servings from a variety of foods chosen from *all* the food groups. That way you get the essential nutrients. Use the following chart to help you see whether your diet is well balanced.

If you're like many other American adults, you tend to eat too many servings of whole-milk dairy products and fatty meats. You probably also eat too few low-fat foods, such as breads, cereals, pasta, vegetables, and fruits. Your good health depends on your eating a balanced diet every day. Choose a variety of nonfat and low-fat foods from each category.

♡ A Change of Diet, a Change of Heart

When you reduce the amount and kinds of fat you eat, you'll gain many significant health benefits. You

How to Create a Balanced Diet

Food category	Recommended number of servings*	The number of servings I usually eat each day is (choose only one):		
		Too Few	Right On	Too Many
Breads, Cereals, Pasta, and Starchy Vegetables	6 or more per day	❑	❑	❑
Vegetables and Fruits	5 or more per day	❑	❑	❑
Skim Milk and Low-Fat Dairy Products	2 to 4 for adults over 24 and children 2 to 10; 3 to 4 for ages 11 to 24 and women who are pregnant or breast-feeding	❑	❑	❑
Lean Meat, Poultry, Seafood, and Eggs	2 servings (no more than a total of 6 oz of cooked poultry, seafood, or lean meat per day)	❑	❑	❑
	No more than 3 or 4 egg yolks per week	❑	❑	❑
Now and Then—Foods from the Tip of the Pyramid	Use sparingly		❑	❑

---

*One serving is equal to:

*Breads, Cereals, Pasta,
and Starchy Vegetables*
1 slice of bread
¼ cup nugget-type cereal
½ cup hot cereal
1 cup ready-to-eat cereal
1 cup cooked rice or pasta
¼ to ½ cup starchy
    vegetables

Vegetables and Fruits

½ cup to 1 cup cooked or
    raw nonstarchy vegetables
    or fruits
1 medium-size piece of fruit
½ cup juice

*Skim Milk and Low-Fat
Dairy Products*
1 cup nonfat or low-fat milk
    or yogurt
1 oz nonfat or low-fat
    hard cheese
½ cup low-fat soft cheese
    (e.g., cottage cheese)

*Lean Meat, Poultry,
Seafood, and Eggs*
3 oz cooked (4 oz raw)
    meat, poultry, or seafood
    (about the size of a deck
    of cards)

---

might lose some extra weight and lower your blood cholesterol level, thus reducing your risk of heart attack and stroke. But changing lifelong eating habits will require effort and commitment on your part. The following tips can make this process a little easier.

Do Only What You're Ready to Do

The Food Diary on page 6 gave you an idea of what you eat. For example, you may have found that you eat very few vegetables and no fruits. You may not be ready to start eating fruit. But you may be willing to try eating more vegetables.

The "Fat IQ" quiz on page 24 showed which areas of your diet could use some "fat-tuning." For example, you may have found that whole-milk cheeses are a significant source of fat, saturated fat, and cholesterol in your diet. But you may not feel ready to change your cheese-eating habits right now. That's okay. Find another habit or food choice that you *are* willing to change today and focus on that. You can always work on your cheese intake later.

The "How to Create a Balanced Diet" chart on pages 28 and 29 helped you see whether your diet is balanced. Maybe you don't get enough dairy products because you don't like to drink milk. But maybe you'd be willing to eat one of the new flavors of non-fat or low-fat yogurt for a snack for a few days. We've tried to give you several ideas to help you make a change. Please do *something*. If you procrastinate and do nothing, you'll never be able to reduce your risk of heart attack. Instead, plan your changes (see page 33). Start with a few simple fat-busting ideas that you can do right now.

Don't Try to Change Everything at Once

Trying to revamp your entire diet at one time can be overwhelming. The truth is, you're more likely to stick with your changes if you tackle them a few at a time. Focus on making one or two changes until they become a habit. Then pick one or two new things to change. You'll discover that many skills you use to make the easy changes will help you succeed in making more-challenging changes later. Over time, you'll reduce the fat in your diet without a great disruption in your daily life. It will simply feel natural.

Easy Does It

It's much easier to take a series of small steps than to make giant leaps. When you make drastic changes, your tastebuds don't have time to adjust to the new flavors and textures that come with low-fat eating. You also need time to practice new skills, such as ordering a heart-healthy meal at a restaurant or learning low-fat ways to prepare vegetables. The changes in this book are designed to help you cut fat, saturated fat, and cholesterol slowly but surely. The key? Easy does it.

Slips Happen

So you had a slice of Italian cream cake at the office party. Just know up front that holidays, special occasions, and illness can distract you from your dietary-change goals. That's okay. Lapses will happen, so don't get down on yourself. Instead, try to figure out what triggered the slip. Then plan ways to avoid that trigger. Sometimes planning ahead is all you need to do to prevent lapses. For example, special occasions don't have to be a problem. We'll show you dozens of fat-busting tips that work for all your meals. You *can* enjoy your food and still do your heart good.

With a Little Help from Your Friends

Any family member over the age of two can enjoy (and benefit from) a low-fat diet. In fact, it's the natural way of eating. You might even ask friends to join you and compare fat-busting notes. It's easier to make and maintain changes when you're surrounded by people who support your efforts.

Think Positive

Please notice: *This book doesn't tell you what you can't eat.* Instead, it introduces you to a world of mouthwatering heart-healthy foods. It's packed with easy ideas for making low-fat foods a part of your everyday life. And it shows you how to reduce your fat intake yet still enjoy your favorite foods—in moderation.

Taste Is a Matter of Taste

If you're used to drinking whole milk, the idea of drinking skim milk may not appeal to you. But trust us. Many people who have switched to 1% milk or skim milk can no longer tolerate the taste of whole milk, claiming that it's too rich or tastes spoiled. Likewise, if you start eating lean ground beef and low-fat cheese, you may begin to favor them. In time, you may prefer a low-fat diet to one full of rich, fatty foods. You'll become hooked on flavor, not fat.

Getting Your Just Rewards

Changing your eating habits takes work. Begin by "Planning for Change" (see page 33). Then, when you've achieved your goals, reward yourself with a nonfood treat! Think of rewards as anything you enjoy but don't get to do or to have often. For example, take an afternoon hike at a nearby park, see a

movie, or buy a new outfit or a CD by your favorite
singer. You are limited only by your imagination.

Planning for Change

1. Review your "Food Diary" on pages 6 and 7, the "Fat IQ"
quiz on pages 12–24, and "How to Create a Balanced Diet"
on pages 28 and 29. List your current high-fat eating
habits below.

_____

_____

_____

_____

2. Circle one or two habits you are willing to change *right
now*. Don't circle more than two.

3. In the space below, map strategies you can use to change
your selected habit(s). Read this book for other ideas and
hints that will help you accomplish your goals.

	Dates	Strategies
Week 1	(_____ to _____)	_____
Week 2	(_____ to _____)	_____
Week 3	(_____ to _____)	_____
Week 4	(_____ to _____)	_____
Week 5	(_____ to _____)	_____
Week 6	(_____ to _____)	_____

I will reward myself by _____

_____

Date _____

An Easy Takeoff

Are you ready to begin your six-week fat-fighting game plan? Great! Let's get started. This week, we'll focus on *easy* ways to start trimming the fat, saturated fat, and cholesterol from your diet—without compromising convenience or flavor.

When lowering your fat intake, it's important to cut back on saturated fat. That will give you the best results in lowering your blood cholesterol and reducing your risk of heart disease. Remember also that "low fat" doesn't always mean "low calorie." Almost any food has too many calories if you eat too much of it.

You'll learn how to substitute low-fat alternatives for high-fat ingredients in recipes. You'll also learn how to make smart choices at restaurants and at the grocery store. And you'll learn that you don't have to give up your favorite foods. We'll show you how to have your burger—and eat it, too!

You may want to read through this entire chapter, or maybe you'd rather just review the one or two food groups that cause you the most trouble. Choose the strategies you think will work best, then practice them for a while. You'll find that some will be easier to master than others, but don't give up on the harder ones. You didn't acquire your old eating habits in a week, so you probably won't create new ones in a week either. When you have mastered a strategy, put a check mark in the box next to it. Try to make at least one check mark each day. Every check mark you make represents progress. At the end of the week, take a look at how you did. If you're ready, go on to the next week, and so on. If you want to go back through this chapter, that's fine. Remember, you can use this book as a basis for a program suited to *your* pace and needs. Just don't tackle so many tips at once that you feel overloaded and give up. The idea is to make changes that can become second nature. If you skip a few things, don't worry. You can always come back later and do them.

♡ Breads, Cereals, Pasta, and Starchy Vegetables

This group is the foundation of a good eating plan. In fact, the Healthy Heart Food Pyramid on page xi is built on a solid foundation of starchy foods. There are many kinds to choose from, and they fill you up wonderfully. Just look at the selections in the list on page 36.

Starchy Foods

Breads	Lentils	Potatoes
Cereals	Lima beans	Rice
Corn	Pasta	Sweet potatoes
Dried beans	Peas	Winter squash

According to popular myth, starchy foods, such as breads, rice, and pasta, are fattening. But that's not true. Most—but not all—starches are low in fat and easy on the heart. It's the butter, cream sauces, pestos, and other high-fat condiments typically added to starch dishes that get you in trouble. This week, let's concentrate on making low-fat selections from this food group.

Bread Winners

❑ Limit croissants, corn bread, quick breads, muffins, biscuits, high-fat crackers, and flour tortillas. You'd be surprised at how much hidden fat these foods often contain. (See the chart on page 37. Our charts refer to grams [g] of fat and saturated fat and to milligrams [mg] of cholesterol.)

Labels, Labels, Labels

When you buy a bread product, look at the easy-to-read food labels. They tell you just how much fat and saturated fat are in one serving. You may be in for a few surprises.

❑ Select breads and crackers that have no more than 2 grams of fat per serving. You'll find plenty to choose from in this category (see page 38).

❑ Choose cereals with fewer than 3 grams of fat per serving. Read the label when it comes to granola-type cereals. They sound healthful, but don't be fooled. Many granola cereals pack more than 275 calories and an astounding 15 grams of fat in a ½-cup serving.

❑ Feel free to fill up on pasta. If you don't top it with cream sauce or pesto, it's naturally low in fat.

❑ Instead of egg noodles, try "eggless" noodles. This will save you about 1.5 grams of fat per cup.

❑ Leave the butter out when you prepare packaged pasta and rice mix recipes.

Bread and Butter: A Look at High-Fat Breads and Bread Products

	Calories	Fat (g)
Croissant (1 medium)	235	12
Biscuit (3″ diameter)	191	7
Corn bread (3 ¼″ x 2 ½″ piece)	189	6
Bran muffin (1)	112	5
Cheese crackers (5)	81	5
Blueberry muffin (1)	126	4
Flour tortilla (8″ diameter)	110	3
Quick bread (2-oz slice)	197	2

Breads for Life: A Better Bet for Your Heart

A serving of each of the following foods (see page 57 for serving sizes) contains only about 80 calories and 1 gram or less of fat and, therefore, a minimum of saturated fat:

Corn tortillas	Low-fat whole-grain crackers
English muffin	Pita
Fat-free muffin	Pumpernickel bread
French bread	Rye bread
Italian bread	Sourdough bread
Low-fat flour tortillas	Whole-wheat bread

♡ Vegetables and Fruits

Vegetables and fruits are naturally low in fat. (The one exception is avocados.) It's too bad that we often hide the bountiful goodness of vegetables and fruits under thick blankets of breading, cheese, cream sauce, or whipped cream. The following tips will help you stay on the low-fat track with fruits and vegetables.

Smart Choices

❑ You don't have to drown a healthful salad with a high-fat dressing. Choose nonfat or low-fat dress-

ings. Spread your wings and give fruit vinegars a
try. Most grocery stores stock raspberry, strawberry, and other sweet, light vinegars.

❑ When choosing frozen or canned vegetables,
go for the ones without added salt or fatty
sauces.

❑ Go easy on fried vegetables.

❑ Order double vegetables instead of double
cheese on your pizza.

❑ Desserts are some of the biggest fat and cholesterol offenders. Try your hand at creating some
low-fat desserts. For instance, fruit with a nonfat
or low-fat topping, such as vanilla yogurt, might
tingle your tastebuds.

❑ For the best nutritional and economic value when
choosing fresh fruits and vegetables, buy them in
season.

Fat-Fighting Facts

◆ Eating a salad is a great way to get part of your
daily fruit and vegetable quota. But when you're eating from a salad bar, you have to know what to put
on your plate and what to pass up. Otherwise, what
starts as a low-fat salad may become buried under
high-fat additions such as excess dressing, croutons, nuts, and cheese. Take a look at the chart on
page 40 for some suggestions for your next trip to
the salad bar.

Choose a Salad That Works— More or Less

Use More . . .		Use Less . . .
◆ Artichoke hearts	◆ Egg whites	◆ Bacon bits
◆ Asparagus	◆ Grapes	◆ Cheese
◆ Bean sprouts	◆ Green peas	◆ Coleslaw
◆ Beans (kidney, pinto, chick-peas, etc.) without dressings or high-fat marinades	◆ Leafy greens (remember, the darker the green, the better)	◆ Croutons
		◆ Egg yolks
		◆ Fried Chinese noodles
	◆ Melon	◆ Macaroni salad
◆ Beets	◆ Mushrooms	◆ Marinated salads
◆ Broccoli	◆ Peppers	◆ Nuts
◆ Cabbage	◆ Pineapple	◆ Olives
◆ Carrots	◆ Raisins	◆ Potato salad
◆ Cauliflower	◆ Squash	◆ Sunflower seeds
◆ Celery	◆ Strawberries	
◆ Cucumber	◆ Tomatoes	
	◆ Water chestnuts	
	◆ Watermelon	

Salad Bar Sabotage

One study showed that college students who ate a hot dinner consumed fewer calories and less fat than did students who ate at the "healthy" salad bar.

The Freshness Quest

Are fresh fruits and vegetables best for you? It depends. If you have time to rinse, peel, and slice them, sure. But if you're short on time or if your produce is going to languish in your refrigerator for weeks, we'd say no. Instead, choose frozen, canned, or dried fruits and vegetables. They're quick and easy. The idea is to *eat* fruits and vegetables—not let them sit in the fridge.

◆ Frozen—Choose the types that don't have added fat (such as cheese or cream sauces), salt, or sugar.

◆ Canned—Choose vegetables without added salt and fruit packed in water or juice. If you want to reduce the sodium content, rinse canned vegetables briefly in a colander or strainer.

◆ Dried—Watch out for sugar and chocolate coatings. Also, remember that dried fruit is a concentrated source of calories.

♡ *Skim Milk and Low-Fat Dairy Products*

Milk, yogurt, and cheese are excellent sources of calcium. But you can also get a hefty dose of fat—especially saturated fat—if you're not careful. The following tips will help you take a big bite out of the fat that comes from dairy products.

How to Milk Dairy Products for All They're Worth

❑ You may not be ready to make the switch from whole to skim milk in one giant leap. Instead, drink 2% milk for a week or two. Then drink 1% for the next week or so. Then switch to skim milk. You'll be glad you did.

❑ Not all yogurt is created equal. Some is made from whole milk. Read the label and choose yogurts made with nonfat or 1% milk. Or look for yogurts that have no more than 3 grams of fat per 8-ounce (1-cup) serving.

❑ Pass the cheese, please—as long as it's nonfat or low-fat. Many people think of cheese as "health food." True, it's a good source of calcium. But an ounce of hard cheese, such as Cheddar, can have about 9 grams of fat and 5 grams of saturated fat! By contrast, low-fat Cheddar has about 5 grams of fat and 3 grams of saturated fat. And nonfat Cheddar doesn't have any! So gradually switch to the healthful cheese choices now available.

❑ You don't have to give up frozen desserts to cut fat. Try ice milk, nonfat or low-fat ice cream, or nonfat or low-fat frozen yogurt. These lower-fat versions can save you as much as 26 grams of fat per ½-cup serving compared with regular ice cream. And they come in flavors just as tantalizing as the rich gourmet ice creams.

Chewing the Fat about Milk

What type of milk are you currently buying? Look at the chart on page 43 to see how much fat and cholesterol and how many calories you can save every year by switching to a lower-fat milk (if you drink 2 cups of milk a day). That's a great savings.

Consider this: you gain one pound for every 3,500 extra calories you eat.

The Straight Skinny on Milk

Different types of milk may look the same, but they're not at all! Fat content varies widely.

One Cup (8 oz)	Total Fat (g)	Saturated Fat (g)	Cholesterol (mg)	Calories
Whole milk	8.2	5.1	33	150
2% milk	4.7	2.9	18	121
1% milk	2.6	1.6	10	102
Skim milk	0.4	0.3	4	86

Fat-Fighting Facts

◆ Whole milk, 2% milk, cheese, and ice cream are major sources of saturated fat in the American diet.

◆ The label might read "2% *low-fat* milk," but don't be fooled. It still has nearly 5 grams of fat and almost 3 grams of

Fat Chance

Current Choice	Change To	Savings per Year			
		Total Fat (g)	Saturated Fat (g)	Cholesterol (mg)	Calories
Whole milk	2%	2,555	1,606	10,950	21,170
Whole milk	1%	4,088	2,555	16,790	34,950
Whole milk	Skim	5,694	3,504	21,170	46,720
2% milk	1%	1,533	949	5,840	13,780
2% milk	Skim	3,139	1,898	10,220	25,550
1% milk	Skim	1,606	949	2,820	11,680

Low-Fat Fact

Both low-fat and nonfat milk have all the nutrients (calcium, vitamins A and D, riboflavin) of regular milk but with little or no fat.

saturated fat per 8-ounce serving. If you're drinking the recommended two to three servings of milk each day, you're getting 2 to 3 teaspoons of fat along with your milk!

◆ If you're now drinking 1% milk, congratulations! It truly is low-fat milk. But if you drink a lot of milk, you may want to consider gradually switching to skim.

◆ Buttermilk made with skim milk is a low-fat alternative to whole milk.

◆ Cream cheese is just that—cheese made from cream. So it's loaded with fat and saturated fat. But don't despair— your bagel need not be plain. Today's dairy cases hold many types of light or nonfat cream cheese.

◆ You can't see the fat in cheese, but it's there. Take a look at the chart on page 45.

◆ One-half cup of premium ice cream can have as much as 26 grams of fat, most of that saturated.

Milk Is IN—Fat Is OUT

In the old days, dairy products were made only from whole milk. But consumer demand for nonfat and low-fat products has radically changed our dairy counters. Now you can buy nonfat and low-fat milk, cheese, yogurt, and ice cream. If your grocery store

Be a Cheese Whiz!

Cheese Type	Amount	Total Fat (g)	Saturated Fat (g)	Cholesterol (mg)	Calories
American	1 oz	8.9	5.6	27	106
Brie	1 oz	7.9	5.3	28	95
Cheddar	1 oz	9.4	6.0	30	114
Colby	1 oz	9.1	5.7	27	112
Cottage (4% milkfat)	½ cup	4.3	3.0	16	109
Cottage (1% milkfat)	½ cup	1.2	0.7	5	82
Cream	2 tbsp	9.9	6.2	31	99
Monterey Jack	1 oz	9.0	5.0	20	110
Mozzarella (part-skim)	1 oz	4.5	2.9	16	72
Muenster	1 oz	8.5	5.4	27	104
Ricotta (part-skim)	½ cup	9.8	6.1	38	171
Swiss	1 oz	7.8	5.0	26	107

doesn't carry the nonfat or low-fat dairy products
you want, talk to the manager about adding them or
shop elsewhere. It's *that* important.

 ## Lean Meat, Poultry, Seafood, and Eggs

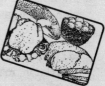

Foods in this group are the source of most of the fat
in the American diet. You can make a big difference

by choosing chicken, turkey, seafood, and lean cuts of beef and pork. Here are some ideas to get you started.

Don't Eat the Fatted Calf

❑ If you're a meat eater, choose from the many varieties of lean meat that are available (see chart on page 49).

❑ Choose ground beef carefully. In some cases, fat is added when the beef is ground. When buying ground beef, choose packages labeled "lean," "extra lean," "10% fat," "90% lean," "5% fat," or "95% lean."

❑ Choose ground turkey made from the *breast only* and ground without the skin. That kind of ground turkey is extremely lean. However, stores sometimes add skin and fat to ground turkey, making it just as fatty as regular ground beef. If in doubt, check with your butcher.

❑ Like the taste of beef? Mix equal parts of lean ground beef with ground skinless turkey *breast*. This mixture gives you the flavor of beef but with less fat.

❑ Eat poultry without the skin, which is relatively high in saturated fat.

❑ Eat fish a few times a week. In general, fish is low in fat, especially saturated fat. Some types, such as salmon, mackerel, and herring, are fairly high in fat. But the *type* of fat in these fish is better for you than the fat in meat and poultry. As a rule, any kind of fish is always a good choice.

❑ Try egg substitutes. They're made from egg whites, a little bit of vegetable oil, and some flavorings. They look like whole eggs, they taste like whole eggs, but they're easier on your heart than the real thing.

Fat-Fighting Facts

◆ Prime, Choice, or Select? That is the question. Meats are graded by fat content. Prime cuts have the most fat. Then comes Choice. Select cuts are the leanest. Next time you're at the meat case, select Select.

◆ Foods in the meat case are not always labeled. Ask the butcher for the leanest cuts.

◆ White meat of poultry has less fat than dark meat.

◆ Don't go "a fowl" with poultry. Goose and duck are higher in fat and saturated fat than chicken, turkey, and Cornish hens.

◆ Pork has been compared with chicken as another source of "white meat." Indeed, many cuts of pork are very lean (see list on page 49). But other light-colored cuts of pork are high in fat. Check with your butcher about which cuts are lowest in fat.

◆ Bacon is really a fat, not a meat. That's because cooked bacon has nearly twice as many fat grams as protein grams. Try the leaner Canadian bacon or lean ham instead.

◆ Turkey bacon and bacon made from soy products have about half the fat and a lot less saturated fat than pork bacon.

◆ Sausage is another high-fat breakfast meat. Look for packages labeled "reduced fat." Keep in mind that even reduced-fat sausage patties and links can still be fairly high in fat. Check the nutrition label.

◆ Low-fat bologna isn't a bunch of boloney. In the old days, bologna and other high-fat items were the most popular luncheon meats. Now you can find tons of low-fat alternatives to choose from. The chart on page 49 lists some of them.

◆ Food manufacturers have not come up with low-fat versions of bratwurst, liverwurst, or salami. So go easy on these foods.

What's the Beef?

Ground beef is one of the biggest sources of fat and saturated fat in the average diet.

Cholesterol Quiz

Which has more cholesterol—3 ounces of skinless chicken breast or 3 ounces of lean beef? Beef, right? Wrong! It's a trick question. Each contains about 70 milligrams of cholesterol. But skinless chicken breast has less fat and saturated fat than lean beef.

Hot Diggity Dog

Regular beef and pork hot dogs are more like sausages. Each hot dog can have as many as 16 grams of fat! Turkey and chicken franks have a little less fat. But no matter which you choose, you're better off with hot dogs labeled "fat free" or "low fat."

Lean and Mean: Looking for the Kindest Cuts

Beef	Pork	Sandwich Meats
Eye of round	Tenderloin	Chicken breast
Top round steak	Sirloin chop	Turkey breast
Tip round roast	Loin roast	Fat-free bologna
Sirloin steak	Top loin chop	Lean ham and roast beef
Top loin steak	Loin chop	Turkey pastrami
Tenderloin steak	Rib chop	
Flank steak	Rib roast	
	Sirloin roast	

♡ Now and Then— Foods from the Tip of the Pyramid

This group contains everything not in the rest of the Healthy Heart Food Pyramid, including fats, oils, salad dressings, sweets, nuts, and snack-type foods.

About 70% of Americans think they have to eliminate their favorite foods to eat a healthful diet. But

Shrimp Is Back on the Low-Fat Track

That's right. Shrimp and crayfish are on the heart-healthy menu again! Many people had banished them because of their high cholesterol content. They're low in total fat and saturated fat, however, so you can eat shrimp and crayfish in moderation.

that's not true. The low-fat message does *not* mean
doom and gloom. Any food can fit into a *6 Weeks to
Get Out the Fat* eating plan. All you have to do is
choose low-fat foods most of the time. Good nutrition is simply knowing what to eat and how much to
eat (this is the topic of Week 2). Then put that knowledge to work for you consistently. That means 80%
or more of the time.

This week we're going to focus on selecting fats,
salad dressings, and sweets. Some fairly simple
approaches can *Get Out the Fat* in a big way.

Fats, Dressings, and Sweets

❑ Use tub margarine rather than stick margarine or
butter.

❑ Use less margarine.

❑ Try butter-flavored spray and granules to add
butter flavor to foods without adding fat.

❑ Salad dressings contribute significantly to the
overall fat in the American diet. Regular salad
dressings contain 55 to 100 calories and 6 to 10
grams of fat per tablespoon. Choose nonfat or
low-fat varieties when possible (see chart on
page 51).

❑ A typical salad dressing ladle holds 4 tablespoons! Learn to enjoy the different flavors and
textures of the salad itself, and use dressings
sparingly.

❑ Most vinaigrette salad dressings are three parts oil
and one part vinegar. To reduce oil in salad dress-

ings of this type, replace some of it with fruit juice concentrates or broth thickened with cornstarch. Or use more of a mild vinegar, such as balsamic.

❑ If you have a sweet tooth and tend to gravitate to high-fat desserts, determine your definition of "moderation." The truth is, you can still enjoy these splurges—just limit them to once a week or once a month.

❑ Cutting your fat intake doesn't mean giving up dessert! Simply choose desserts with little or no fat (see chart on page 53).

Butter or Margarine?

Although both butter and margarine are fat, butter has cholesterol and is much higher in saturated fat. So choose margarine instead of butter.

Dressing for Success

Salad Dressing (1 tbsp)	Calories	Fat (g)
Fat-free dressing	5–25	0
Lemon juice	0	0
Picante sauce	4	0
Balsamic vinegar	6	0
Fruit vinegars	6	0
Reduced-calorie dressing, all types	15–40	2–4
Nonfat mayonnaise	12	0
Reduced-fat mayonnaise	50	5

How to Make a Big Fat Difference

	Calories	Fat (g)	Saturated Fat (g)	Cholesterol (mg)	Sodium (mg)
Butter (1 tbsp)	100	11	7	30	85
Whipped butter (1 tbsp)	60	7	5	20	75
Stick margarine (1 tbsp)	90	10	2	0	110
Tub margarine (1 tbsp)	80	9	1.5	0	90
Light tub margarine (1 tbsp)	40	4.5	0	0	90
Squeeze margarine (1 tbsp)	80	9	1.5	0	100
Butter-flavored spray (5 sprays)	0	0	0	0	0
Butter-flavored granules (1 tsp)	5	0	0	0	45

Low-Fat Treats

- Angel food cake topped with slightly sweetened sliced berries
- Baked apple with a dash of cinnamon
- Dried fruits
- Fig and other fruit bars
- Fresh fruit bowl
- Frozen fruit juice bars
- Frozen yogurt
- Gingersnaps
- Graham crackers
- Hard candy
- Italian ice
- Jelly beans
- Low-fat and nonfat baked goods
- Poached pears with raspberry sauce
- Pudding made with nonfat or low-fat milk
- Sherbet
- Sorbet
- Vanilla wafers
- Warm fruit compote

Eating Out—Eating Healthy

You can eat out without going overboard on fat. In fact, about 40% of U.S. restaurants now offer healthful menu selections lower in fat, saturated fat, cholesterol, sodium, and calories. If you eat out often, plan ahead. This advanced planning can help you make healthful menu selections and prevent the day's circumstances, your moods, your environment, and other distractions from interfering with your good intentions.

A Frequent Diner's Guide to Help-Your-Heart Eating

❏ Choose restaurants that you know have heart-healthy options.

❏ Decide what you're going to have before you get to the restaurant.

❏ Be the first to order, if possible. This helps prevent temptation.

❏ Ask the waiter to leave potato chips, fries, and other high-fat items off your plate.

❏ Make sure your meal includes a serving of fruit or a vegetable. Better yet, order one of each.

❏ Begin your meal with water and salad, raw vegetables, or clear soup. Or start with a snack like this at home before you leave for the restaurant.

❏ Select a soup or salad that's low in fat (see chart on page 55).

❏ Beware of prebuttered bread and rolls with a glaze. These fats add up. Ask for plain bread or a plain roll instead.

❏ When selecting an entrée, look for poultry, seafood, or lean cuts of beef, such as filet, top sirloin, flank steak, London broil, or shish kebab.

Make It or Break It with Soups and Salads

SOUP

Lentil
Manhattan clam chowder
Minestrone
Onion soup without the
  bread and cheese
Potato leek
Split pea
Vegetable

SALAD

Chick-peas and kidney
  beans
Fresh vegetables
Fruit
Lemon juice instead of
  dressing
Low-fat and low-calorie
  dressings
Oil and vinegar

SOUP

Cream-based soups
New England
  clam chowder

SALAD

Avocado
Bacon bits
Butter-fried croutons
Cheese
Chicken and tuna salad
  made with mayonnaise
Eggs
Marinated vegetables
Meats

Eating the **R**ight **A**mount

Congratulations! You're ready to begin your second week of the *6 Weeks to Get Out the Fat* program. This week, you'll learn that good nutrition is knowing how much to eat, as well as what to eat. Eating the correct amount from each food group each day will help you reduce your fat intake.

Today food manufacturers give us many products that are low in fat. These products include salad dressings, baked goods, frozen desserts, and dozens more. Remember, "low fat" doesn't necessarily mean "low calorie." In fact, some low-fat foods are as high in calories as the original high-fat version. That's why it's still important to control how much you eat.

To start, you may want to concentrate your efforts on the food group that gives you the most trouble— whether you may be eating too much or not enough of it. Look for strategies and ideas that will work best for you. As you put them into play in your fat-cutting program, mark them with a check.

♡ Breads, Cereals, Pasta, and Starchy Vegetables

In Week 1 you learned that this food group is the foundation of a healthful eating plan. Nutritionists recommend eating six *or more* servings each day from this food group. Sounds like the sky's the limit, right? Not really. Although the foods in this group are naturally low in fat and relatively low in calories, you can still add unwanted weight if you pig out.

Frankly, it's easy to overeat from this food group because so many restaurants serve gargantuan portions of breads and pastas. Also, in recent years, oversized bagels and muffins have become the rage. That's why it's important to clarify how much of each food constitutes a *normal* serving and how many servings a day are best. Take a look at the chart below for some *typical* household serving sizes from this group. (The serving sizes of some packaged foods may differ slightly from these serving sizes. You can estimate the nutrient content of different serving sizes by comparing the values given on the labels.)

What Is a Serving, Anyway?

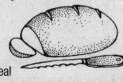

- ◆ 1 slice of bread
- ◆ ⅓–½ bagel
- ◆ 1 cup of cooked rice or pasta
- ◆ 1 cup of flaked cereal
- ◆ ¼ cup of nugget or bud-type cereal
- ◆ ½ cup of cooked cereal
- ◆ ¼–½ cup of starchy vegetables

Recommended Number of Servings

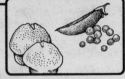

Preschool children ▬ **4 servings**

Preadolescents ▬▬▬ **4 or more servings**

Adolescents ▬▬▬▬ **6 or more servings**

Adults ▬▬▬▬ **6 or more servings**

How Many Servings Do You Need Each Day?

Although the number of servings you need varies
with your activity level, you can use the above chart
as a guide.

Starchy Food Rules

❑ Keep track of how many servings from this group
you eat during the day. You may be surprised at
how easily they add up.

❑ Serve yourself reasonable portions of pasta and
rice (see chart on page 57).

❑ Request a small or medium baked potato rather
than a potato the size of Idaho.

❑ If dinner rolls around and you've already eaten
your starch allotment, skip the bread, pasta, rice,
or potato. Eat a double serving of steamed vegetables instead.

❑ Count your crackers. A serving is not the whole
box. Read the label and munch accordingly.

Food for Thought

A serving is not necessarily what you serve yourself. Look carefully at the chart on page 57. Compare those amounts with the portions you usually eat. You may need to make some adjustments.

*R*eality Check

1 bagel could be 2–3 servings.

A "bowl" of cereal could be 2–4 servings.

A burrito-size tortilla could be 2 servings.

A restaurant portion of pasta could be 3–6 servings.

♡ *Vegetables and Fruits*

If you're like many other Americans, you probably don't eat enough vegetables and fruits each day. And if you're shortchanging yourself here, you could be missing out on important nutrients, such as dietary fiber and vitamins A and C. The following tips will help you make eating vegetables and fruits a healthful habit.

Broccoli, Anyone?

❑ You don't have to eat a whole orchard to meet your fruit and vegetable requirement. Just eat five or more servings a day.

❑ Keep serving sizes in mind (see chart on page 60).

What Is a Serving, Anyway?

- ◆ 1 medium piece of fruit
- ◆ ½–1 cup cooked or raw vegetables
- ◆ ½ cup fruit or vegetable juice

❑ Try to have at least one fruit and/or vegetable serving at every meal—even if it's just a glass of juice.

❑ If you're bored with the same old steamed broccoli or canned fruit cocktail, you may not reach your "five-a-day" goal. Put some punch in your diet by eating veggie mixtures, trying new fruits, or exploring new nonfat or low-fat toppings.

❑ Put fruit instead of butter or margarine on toast. Try apple butter, all-fruit spreads, even sliced fresh bananas or strawberries.

❑ Don't worry if you don't get all five of your fruit and vegetable servings *every* single day. Try to eat an average of five servings per day over the course of a week.

Fixing Tricks

Think fitting fruits and vegetables into your everyday life is a hassle? Here are some tricks that may make it easier for you to get your daily quota.

- ◆ Use fruits and vegetables as low-fat snacks.
- ◆ Shop for fruits and vegetables on the weekend. At home, spend a little time cutting them up and storing them in containers and plastic bags so they'll be convenient.

◆ Buy precut veggies.

◆ Try premade green salads. Be sure to choose the ones packaged with low-fat or nonfat dressings, or use your own fat-free dressings.

◆ Drink your fruits and veggies. You'll get all the nutrition (except some of the fiber) without having to peel, slice, and chop. Remember, there's more to juice than just orange juice! Be an explorer: Try tomato, grapefruit, apricot, or carrot juice.

𝕸issing in Action

The average American only eats 3½ servings of fruits and vegetables per day. That's 548 missing servings per person per year!

Keep a weekly fruit and vegetable scorecard (see pages 62 and 63). Carry it in your pocket or purse. At each meal or snack time, check one box on your scorecard for each serving of fruits and vegetables you eat. Remember, your goal is to eat at least five servings of fruits and/or vegetables each day. As you get better at it, you can keep score in your head.

Dollars and Nutrition Sense

Many people think fruits and vegetables are expensive. But take another look. The chart on page 64 shows you which foods give you more nutritional bang for your buck.

Vegetables and Fruits Daily Scorecard

To help you keep track of your vegetable and fruit
intake, put a check (4) in the appropriate box each time
you eat a vegetable or fruit serving. If you aren't quite
reaching your goal of at least five servings of vegetables
and fruits a day, look for ways to boost your score.

Day of Week	Vegetables				
SUNDAY	❑	❑	❑	❑	❑
MONDAY	❑	❑	❑	❑	❑
TUESDAY	❑	❑	❑	❑	❑
WEDNESDAY	❑	❑	❑	❑	❑
THURSDAY	❑	❑	❑	❑	❑
FRIDAY	❑	❑	❑	❑	❑
SATURDAY	❑	❑	❑	❑	❑

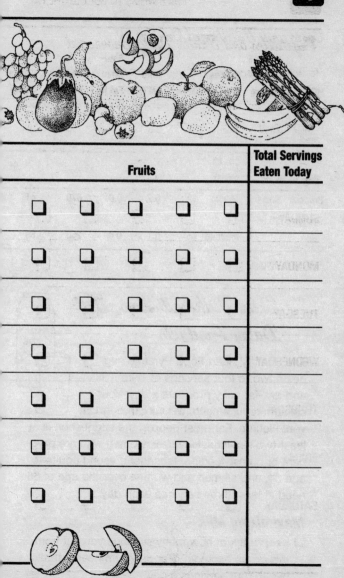

Fruits					Total Servings Eaten Today
❑	❑	❑	❑	❑	
❑	❑	❑	❑	❑	
❑	❑	❑	❑	❑	
❑	❑	❑	❑	❑	
❑	❑	❑	❑	❑	
❑	❑	❑	❑	❑	
❑	❑	❑	❑	❑	

Costs and Nutritional Content

Food	Average Cost per Serving	Serving Size	Calories	Total Fat (g)	Saturated Fat (g)	Vitamin A (IU*)	Vitamin C (mg)
Potato chips	$0.25	1 oz (about 10–12 chips)	152	9.8	3.1	0	9
Broccoli	$0.24	½ cup	12	0.2	0.0	678	41
Orange	$0.35	1 medium	65	0.1	0.0	256	80

*International Units

♡ Skim Milk and Low-Fat Dairy Products

The Healthy Heart Food Pyramid suggests two to four servings of skim milk and low-fat dairy products a day. Your calcium requirements will vary throughout your lifetime. For most people, the suggestion is at least two servings. However, women who are pregnant or breast-feeding, teenagers, young adults to age 24, and all men and women over the age of 65 need at least three servings each day.

Maximizing Milk

❑ Keep track of how many servings you eat from this group each day. For optimum health, that's two to four servings a day.

❑ Keep serving sizes in mind (see chart below).

❑ If you are allergic to milk or are lactose intolerant,
you can try either milk that's lactose free or a
product that helps with milk digestion.

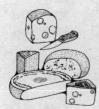

Cheese: Ounce for Ounce

How much is an ounce of cheese?
A cube that measures 1 inch on
each side equals 1 ounce. If it's
shredded cheese, figure about a
quarter-cup. Sliced cheese varies,
depending on the size and thickness of the slice.
Read the label to be sure.

What Is a Serving, Anyway?

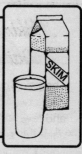

◆ 1 cup of skim or 1% fat milk
◆ 1 cup of nonfat or low-fat yogurt
◆ 1 ounce of nonfat or low-fat cheese
◆ ½ cup of nonfat or low-fat cheese

Calcium Counts—For Life

Your calcium requirements fluctuate with growth
and stage of life. Look at the chart on page 68 to
see how much calcium you need each day. For
instance, you can get about 300 of the needed
milligrams from a cup of skim milk. But you'd have
to eat 2 cups of cottage cheese for an equivalent
amount of calcium.

Calcium Requirements

	mg / day
Birth–6 months	400
Infants (7–12 months)	600
Young children (1–5 years)	800
Older children (6–10 years)	800–1,200
Adolescents and young adults (11–24 years)	1,200–1,500
Women 25–50 years	1,000
Pregnant and breast-feeding women	1,200–1,500
Postmenopausal women on estrogen	1,000
Postmenopausal women not on estrogen	1,500
Men 25–65 years	1,000
All women and men over 65	1,500

♡ *Lean Meat,*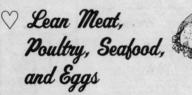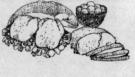
Poultry, Seafood,
and Eggs

Chances are, you get most of your protein from
meat, poultry, and seafood. The problem is, you
probably eat a lot more protein than your body
needs. And unless you're careful, a lot of extra fat,
saturated fat, and cholesterol come with that protein.
Here are a few ideas for cutting your portions along
with your fat, saturated fat, and cholesterol.

Any Way You Slice It, Watch Your Portions

❑ Try to limit yourself to two servings a day from
   this group.

❑ Leave the big packages of meat for big families.
Remember, if you buy less, you'll cook less and
eat less. Or divide the big package into smaller
portions and freeze them.

❑ Avoid eating large patties of ground beef. Instead,
use small amounts of lean ground meat in sauces
(such as spaghetti, taco, and sloppy Joe) and in
casseroles (such as lasagna).

❑ All the fat and cholesterol in eggs is in the yolk.
You can have all the egg whites you want, but
limit your egg yolks to no more than three or four
a week.

❑ Instead of a three-egg omelet, try blending one
whole egg and two or three egg whites. Or use
egg substitute equal to three eggs.

What Is a Serving, Anyway?

◆ 4 ounces raw lean meat (3 ounces cooked)
◆ 4 ounces raw poultry (3 ounces cooked)
◆ 4 ounces raw seafood (3 ounces cooked)

Cutting Your Meat Servings Down to Size

◆ Having trouble keeping your portion sizes to 3 ounces of
cooked meat? A serving is about the size of a deck of
cards. If you want a more precise portion, weigh your food
or ask your butcher to cut your servings down to size.

◆ Expecting meat-hungry guests for dinner? Serve them shish
kebab. It's easy and elegant. You'll dazzle them with your

culinary creativity while keeping meat portions to a minimum.

◆ To be certain about portion sizes, have the deli staff cut your purchase into 1-ounce slices.

◆ Half a chicken breast or a leg and a thigh is about a single serving.

◆ A good way of gauging your portion size of fish is to check the amount in a 3-ounce can of tuna. That's what you need for one serving.

♡ Now and Then—Foods from the Tip of the Pyramid

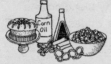 It's not surprising that most Americans love to eat from the "Now and Then" group. The tip of the Healthy Heart Food Pyramid contains fats, oils, nuts, sweets, and basically everything that doesn't fall within one of the other food groups. Although all these foods fit into a healthful eating plan when eaten sparingly, most people have a tendency to overdo—their food pyramids are a bit top-heavy.

Going Easy on Fats and Oils

❑ If you use margarine on breads, rice, pasta, or potatoes, use less. Every teaspoon of margarine contains about 5 grams of fat and 45 calories.

❑ Try the stab method with salad dressings. Dip the tip of your fork into salad dressing and then stab some salad. The objective is to have some salad dressing flavor with every bite but without having your greens drip with dressing.

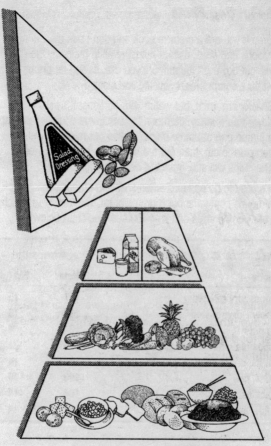

Top-Heavy Food Pyramid

❑ Reduce the amount of nuts in cooking and baking. Better yet, just leave them out.

❑ Consider a mini-portion of dessert or share a dessert with friends. Eat slowly. Enjoy every morsel without feeling deprived.

Fat-Fighting Facts

◆ Even if you are a creative cook and don't use measuring spoons and cups, always measure oil in recipes. Often this will cut down on the amount you use, saving fat grams without compromising quality and taste.

◆ Snacks are great, but watch your portions! It's easy to sit down to a Sunday afternoon football game and casually eat a jumbo bag of potato chips. Portion out how many chips you plan to eat, then put the rest of the bag in the freezer. The chips will stay fresh but be out of sight.

◆ It's easy to go bananas when snacking on nuts. Ten almonds contain about 6 grams of fat. The trick is to watch your portion sizes and limit yourself (see chart below).

Nuts—in a Nutshell

1 Ounce	Calories	Fat (g)
Almonds, dry roasted	167	15
Cashews, dry roasted	163	13
Corn nuts	124	4
Macadamia nuts	199	21
Peanuts, dry roasted	164	14
Pecans, raw	190	19
Pistachios, dried	164	14
Sunflower seeds	162	14

♡ Eating Out—Eating Healthy

When eating out, many people think they're getting value when they get an enormous portion. But huge portions—three or four times the amount in a "normal" serving—can wreak havoc on trying to eat sensibly. The following tips will help you keep portion sizes in the realm of normal when you're eating out.

Oh, Waiter!

❑ If the restaurant gives you a bowl of chips, fried noodles, or nuts, ask the waiter to take it away. Or put a few on your plate and then send the basket away.

❑ A slice of bread or a couple of breadsticks (minus the butter) are good low-fat appetizers. Be careful not to eat everything in the bread basket.

❑ Eat half of an oversized portion or split an entrée. Typically, large steaks, fajitas, pasta entrées, and oriental dishes can easily feed two people. It's a great feeling to leave your favorite restaurant satisfied but not stuffed.

❑ Ask for a carry-out box when you order, and immediately set aside a take-home portion.

Fat-Fighting Facts

◆ Judging portion sizes in a restaurant is important. Try measuring your food at home so you become familiar with portion sizes. That way, when you eat out, you can judge how much to eat.

◆ Remember that 6 ounces of meat is an entire day's supply. (A steak the size of Texas is outside this recommendation!) Ask for the lunch-size portion of meat rather than the dinner-size portion. If that's not available, share your entrée with another person or save part of the meat for another meal.

◆ Dining out can be enjoyable, delicious, and healthy! If you don't throw portion control to the wind, you'll enjoy your dining out experience all the more.

Variety Is the Spice of Life

This week let's keep the momentum going by looking at the need for variety and balance in your eating plan. We all know that eating the same old thing isn't much fun, but it also isn't much good for you. When it comes to nutrition, there's great news. Your body needs more than 40 nutrients to be healthy, and no single food can provide them all. In other words, a healthful eating plan need never be boring.

Healthful eating, like good health itself, is a choice. When it comes to food, you have lots of options. Enjoy these suggestions for putting variety, balance, convenience, and meal planning into your everyday life.

♡ Breads, Cereals, Pasta, and Starchy Vegetables

With so many foods to choose from in this food group, variety and balance should be a snap. At the same time, it's easy to fall into a rut and choose the same starches every day. The challenge is to plan heart-smart, low-fat meals with variety.

Variety Show

❑ Try a low-fat, nutrient-packed hot cereal at lunch or dinner for a change. Piping hot oatmeal, sweetened with raisins or peaches canned in fruit juice . . . Mmm.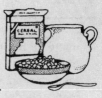

❑ Liven up your breakfast table this week (see the chart on page 74).

❑ Usually eat a sandwich for lunch? Why not try a baked potato instead? Or a baked sweet potato? Or pasta? Get out of that rut!

❑ Try some whole-grain goodness. Experience cereals, breads, pastas, and even waffles made with whole grains. As you strive to eat fewer high-fat foods, whole-grain foods are nutritionally ideal choices. The predominant ingredient should be labeled "whole grain." Look for whole-grain oats, whole-grain wheat, whole-grain rice, whole-grain corn, or whole-grain barley. Also look for "whole wheat," such as whole-wheat flour.

❑ Try brown rice. To cook it, use about 2 cups of water for every 1 cup of raw brown rice. One cup of raw brown rice makes about 3 cups when cooked.

❑ Do some strategic meal planning. All foods can fit into healthful eating—if you have a plan. It's a

Field of Grains

- ◆ Barley
- ◆ Bulgur
- ◆ Couscous
- ◆ Farina
- ◆ Grits (polenta)
- ◆ Millet
- ◆ Oat bran

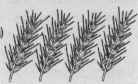

matter of balancing tactics. For example, a piece of corn bread can have as much fat as a piece of fried chicken. If fried chicken is on the picnic menu, choose a yeast roll rather than corn bread.

♡ Vegetables and Fruits

Are frozen vegetables and canned fruit the extent of your culinary capabilities? Here are some fruit and veggie guidelines for a balanced and varied diet.

The Fruit and Veggie Top 20

Breakfast

❑ Top your cereal with fresh, frozen, canned, or dried fruit.

❑ Stir things up with a fruit smoothie. Put fruit and nonfat or low-fat vanilla yogurt in a blender and let it whirl!

❑ Enjoy a glass of cranberry or mixed fruit juice.

❑ Pour pureed fruit over pancakes and waffles.

❑ Add dried fruit when cooking hot cereal.

Lunch

❑ Stash whole pieces of fresh fruit (apple, orange, banana, grapes) in your briefcase, purse, or workout bag.

❑ Order a plateful of steamed veggies.

❑ Pack along leftover fruit salad from last night's dinner.

❑ Make a big dark-green salad with nonfat or low-fat dressing.

❑ Carry a single-serving can of fruit packed in fruit juice.

Dinner

❑ Double or triple up on your vegetables (served with nonfat or low-fat toppings).

❑ Grill green and red bell peppers, cherry tomatoes, zucchini, and onions with your lean steak.

❑ Stir-fry a medley of frozen vegetables.

❑ Dive into a bowl of fresh berries topped with nonfat or low-fat vanilla yogurt.

❑ Core an apple, add a mixture of 1 tablespoon brown sugar and 1/8 teaspoon cinnamon, and bake at 350° F or microwave on high until soft.

Snacks

❑ Carry dried fruit (apples, peaches, prunes, raisins) with you for a quick energy booster.

❑ Dip carrots and other raw veggies into nonfat or low-fat dressing.

❑ Sip on tomato, carrot, or other vegetable juices.

❑ Chill out with frozen fruits (bananas, grapes, strawberries, or cherries).

❑ Buy precut melon at a local market.

*O*range You Glad There's Fruit?

Looking for a low-fat sweet snack? Choose fruit. Think of it as Mother Nature's candy bar.

Eye-Pleasing Meal Planning

Imagine your plate divided in four equal parts. Fill one quarter with starches, one quarter with meat, fish, or poultry, and the last two quarters with fruits and/or veggies. Use different shapes, sizes, and colors to add variety to your fruit and vegetable repertoire (see page 77). Then your food should please your eyes as well as your palate.

Plateful of Vitamins

Fruits and vegetables are packed with nutrients. However, some have more nutrients than others. That's why it's important to eat a variety of fruits and veggies. Each of the foods in the chart on pages 77 and 78 provides at least 25% of your daily requirement of vitamins A and/or C.

Plan for Variety

Shapes	Sizes	Colors
Bell pepper rings	Baby carrots	Blueberries
Carrot coins	Cherry tomatoes	Broccoflower
Julienne zucchini	Jumbo blackberries	Pink grapefruit
Star fruit slices	Pattypan squash	Purple (yes, purple!) potatoes

Vitamins Galore

Vegetables†	Vitamin A	Vitamin C
Asparagus		*
Broccoli	*	*
Brussels sprouts		*
Cabbage		*
Carrots	*	
Cauliflower		*
Green pepper		*
Potato		*
Red leaf lettuce	*	
Romaine lettuce	*	
Salad greens (1 cup raw)	*	*
Spinach	*	*
Sweet potato	*	
Tomato juice	*	*
Tomatoes	*	*
Winter squash	*	
Fruits		
Apricots (3)	*	
Cantaloupe (½ cup)	*	*
Grapefruit (½)		*

(continued on page 78)

Fruits	Vitamin A	Vitamin C
Grapefruit juice (¾ cup)		*
Grapes (1 cup)		*
Honeydew (½ cup)		*
Kiwifruit (1)		*
Nectarine (1)	*	
Orange (1)		*
Orange juice (¾ cup)		*
Papaya (½ cup)	*	*
Raspberries (½ cup)		*
Strawberries (½ cup)		*
Watermelon (1 cup)		*

†Portion size is ½ cup cooked unless otherwise noted.

*Provides at least 25% of your daily requirement of vitamins A and/or C.

Are some of your favorite fruits and veggies missing from the list? Green beans, bananas, apples, pears, and pineapples don't have much vitamin A or C, but they're still good sources of dietary fiber.

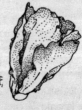

Lettuce Think Green

Many people prefer iceberg to other lettuce. Yet it has hardly any vitamin A, vitamin C, or even dietary fiber. Remember, the greener the leaf, the better.

All Juices Are Not Created Equal

An 8-ounce glass of orange juice has 97 milligrams of vitamin C (one and one-half times your daily requirement) and 112 calories. The same amount of apple juice has *no* vitamin C and 111 calories.

♡ Skim Milk and Low-Fat Dairy Products

You asked for them, you got them!
Manufacturers listened to the demand for nonfat and low-fat dairy products, and now a wide variety is available in the marketplace. Check out the following list for new ideas and variety.

Sacred Cows—Getting the Most Out of Dairy Products

❑ Plan to include nonfat or low-fat milk and other dairy products in your meals to help get the required two to four servings a day.

❑ Try a nonfat or low-fat yogurt flavor that you haven't tasted before.

❑ Try nonfat or low-fat vanilla yogurt mixed with fresh or canned fruit and nugget cereal for breakfast.

❑ If you miss a dairy serving at a meal, try a snack that includes skim milk. Did you know that you can buy nonfat chocolate syrup? Warm or cold, skim milk with chocolate syrup can be a great snack.

❑ If you have access to a refrigerator at work, take a quart of skim milk to keep there. Enjoy a glass of nutrient-packed skim milk rather than an empty-nutrient soft drink with lunch or for a snack!

❑ Keep nonfat dry milk in your cupboard. When reconstituted double strength and served cold, it's delicious. You'll be glad it's on hand when you're out of milk and a pan of low-fat oatmeal cookies has just come out of the oven.

♡ Lean Meat, Poultry, Seafood, and Eggs

Ground beef is America's most popular meat. It's readily available, it's easy to cook, it's versatile, and it tastes good. But there's a lot more to this food group than hamburgers and meat loaf.

Don't Have a Cow—You Don't Need That Much Protein

❑ Treat yourself to new ways of preparing poultry, seafood, and different cuts of meat.

❑ Include fish or other seafood in your meal plans several times this week (see list on page 81 for some suggested varieties).

❑ Skip the meat in a dinner or two this week. Make sure your meatless meals are well-balanced by including

- ◆ nonfat or low-fat starches
- ◆ lots of vegetables and fruits
- ◆ nonfat or low-fat dairy products

Holy Mackerel!

Fishing around for new meal ideas? There are oceans of low-fat seafood options. Even the fattier ones are much lower in saturated fat than most meats.

Seafood Choices

Type*	Total Fat (g)	Saturated Fat (g)	Cholesterol (mg)	Calories
Bass	4.0	0.9	74	124
Clams	1.7	0.2	52	126
Cod	0.7	0.1	47	89
Crab, Alaska king	1.3	0.1	45	82
Crab, blue	1.5	0.2	76	87
Crab, Dungeness	1.1	0.1	64	94
Crayfish	1.2	0.2	151	97
Haddock	0.8	0.1	63	95
Halibut	2.5	0.4	35	119
Herring, Atlantic	9.9	2.2	65	172
Herring, Pacific	15.1	3.5	84	213
Lobster	0.5	0.1	61	83
Mackerel, Atlantic	15.1	3.4	64	223
Mackerel, jack	8.6	2.4	40	171

(continued on page 82)

Type*	Total Fat (g)	Saturated Fat (g)	Cholesterol (mg)	Calories
Mussels	3.8	0.7	48	147
Ocean perch	1.8	0.3	46	103
Orange roughy	0.8	0.0	22	75
Oysters	4.2	1.1	93	117
Pollock	1.1	0.1	77	100
Salmon, Atlantic	6.9	1.1	60	155
Salmon, chinook	11.4	2.7	72	196
Scallops	1.0	0.2	37	88
Sea bass	1.7	0.4	35	82
Shark (3 oz raw)	3.8	0.8	43	111
Shrimp	0.9	0.2	166	84
Snapper	1.5	0.3	40	109
Swordfish	4.4	1.2	43	132
Trout	3.7	0.7	62	100
Tuna	1.1	0.4	51	112

* Portion size is 3 oz cooked weight unless otherwise noted.

Fat-Fighting Facts

◆ Many dishes use meat more as a condiment than as the main ingredient. A little lean meat can go a long way with stir-fries, shish kebabs, stews, soups, and sauces. The flavor options are endless.

◆ When it comes to moderating your portions of meat, don't stew in your own juice. You can get the hearty beef flavor you want by using moist heat and slowly cooking lean cuts of beef for a long time. This method works well for stews and soups. Load them with lots of vitamin-rich vegetables for a variety of flavors.

◆ When making fajitas from poultry or lean skirt or flank steak, save some of the meat to add to a main-dish tossed salad the next day.

♡ *Now and Then—Foods from the Tip of the Pyramid*

 Salty, crunchy, sweet, munchy, smooth, and creamy. It's time for a snack! Believe it or not, snacks can be a part of a healthful and low-fat eating plan. Snacks often come from the tip of the Pyramid. Your challenge is to break out of your regular snack habit and find three or more snacks you don't usually eat. Here are some snacks from other parts of the Pyramid.

Marvelous Munchies

❑ Try a fruit shake. Blend a banana or another fruit with nonfat milk and ice cubes. Stir in a splash of vanilla or a dash of cinnamon.

❑ Mix fruit and/or shredded carrots into flavored gelatin.

❑ Try mixing several kinds of cold cereal for a crunchy snack.

❑ For a rich-tasting snack, put 1 ounce of part-skim mozzarella cheese on melba toast or whole-wheat crackers.

❑ Treat yourself to some hot cocoa made from a nonfat or low-fat mix.

❑ Serve angel food cake with a fresh fruit puree for a refreshing dessert.

❑ Try mixing pretzel pieces and nonfat or low-fat cottage cheese.

Fat-Fighting Facts

◆ Vanilla wafers, graham crackers, animal crackers, ginger-snaps, and fruit bars make good snacks.

◆ Veggie dips don't have to be high in fat. Try salsa for a delightfully different taste.

◆ Frozen veggies that have been partially thawed make interesting snacks. Try corn, peas, or any others that strike your fancy. (Don't knock it 'till you've tried it. Kids love these!)

♡ *Eating Out—Eating Healthy*

It's important to make nutritious choices when eating out. Next time you're at a restaurant, eat with your heart in mind. A simple guideline is to differentiate between *frequent* eating out and *special occasion* eating out.

The average American eats about four meals per week outside the home. About 40% of Americans eat lunch out five to seven times each week! That's a lot. So, if you're trying to *Get Out the Fat,* it's critical to make healthful menu selections when you eat out frequently (see the Eating Out—Eating Healthy sections of Weeks 1 and 2).

On the other hand, dining out on a special occasion can be an appropriate time to eat foods you wouldn't normally choose. Surprised? It's just another way to help you achieve balance and variety in your diet.

Here are some tips for special occasion dining. Give them a try.

Dining Out Tips

☐ Enjoy the company. Talk, talk, talk, and listen, listen, listen.

☐ Eat slowly.

☐ Don't overeat.

☐ Most of all, **enjoy!**

Fat-Fighting Facts

◆ Balance your caloric intake (the food you eat) with your caloric output (the energy you expend). If you eat more than usual, you can balance that by exercising more than usual. For example, take a walk after dinner.

◆ If you overeat at one meal, don't despair. Having your own compensating strategy planned for the next day can help. Know that if you lapse, you'll make up for it with an all-vegetable day, a more exercise day, a mini-meal day, or a two-meal day.

Cooking with Your Heart in Mind

You're halfway to your goal! In Week 1, you tackled the problem of knowing what foods to eat. In Week 2, you focused on determining how much to eat. In Week 3, you learned about eating balanced meals and a variety of foods.

Now, in Week 4, you'll learn how to prepare foods the low-fat, low-cholesterol way. You don't cook? No problem. These pages cover everything from what to spread on bread to how to cook from scratch. And since you're busier than ever these days, we've given top priority to convenience and saving time.

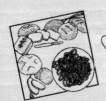

♡ Breads, Cereals, Pasta, and Starchy Vegetables

You already know that most unadorned breads, pasta, and potatoes and other starchy vegetables contain only a trace of fat. But they're rarely left alone. Instead, they're famous for attracting high-fat spreads and toppings. We've listed some better-for-you alternatives below.

Bread Spread

❑ Choose all-fruit jam, jelly, or preserves instead of butter or margarine.

❑ Try nonfat or light cream cheese instead of regular cream cheese on bagels. You may not even notice a difference.

❑ Learn to enjoy the taste of whole-grain breads without a spread.

❑ Try low-fat biscuit and baking mixes. Most people can't tell the difference between foods made with the original mix and those made with the lower-fat version.

Pasta Power

❑ Make your own heart-smart tomato sauce. Buy canned crushed tomatoes. Simmer with minced onion, plenty of garlic, black pepper, and classic Italian herbs, such as basil, oregano, and rosemary. *Bravissimo!*

❑ For other heart-healthy toppings, try fresh vegetables simmered in low-sodium broth with herbs and spices. Top your pasta with these veggies and 1 tablespoon of Parmesan cheese per serving. The cheese adds a mountain of flavor, yet only about 30 calories and less than 3 grams of fat.

Starchy Vegetable Fact and Fiction

❑ Potatoes have a reputation for being fattening, but they aren't. One medium-size baked potato with its skin contains about 220 calories and is virtually fat free. It's the margarine, sour cream, and bacon toppers that do you in. See "Create a Spectacular Spud" on page 89 for some different low-fat toppings.

❑ It's a high-fat fact that a 2½-ounce serving of French fries has nearly 3 times the calories and nearly 12 times the fat as a 2½-ounce baked potato. Make fries a "once-in-a-while" food. For you, that may mean once a week or once a month. You decide what's right for you.

𝑛 ot-So-Hot Tomato Sauce

By far, the most popular topping for pasta is tomato sauce. Read the labels on store-bought sauces. Why? Because some bottled and canned sauces have over 7 grams of fat in a ½-cup serving. Look for one with 3 grams of fat or less instead.

Create a Spectacular Spud

High-Fat Potato Toppers	Low-Fat Potato Toppers
Butter or margarine (12 g per tbsp)	Low-fat salad dressing (0–4 g per tbsp)
Sour cream (2.5 g per tbsp)	Mustard (Dijon, honey, or horseradish style) (0–1 g per tbsp)
Cheddar cheese (9.5 g per ¼ cup)	Light soy sauce (0 g per tbsp)
	Nonfat or low-fat cottage cheese (0–1.1 g per ¼ cup)
	Steak sauce (0 g per tbsp)
	Starchy beans (0.2 g per ¼ cup)
	Salsa (0 g per tbsp)
	Broccoli with reduced-fat cheese melted with skim milk (5 g per ½ cup)

♡ Vegetables and Fruits

Serve them raw or cooked, with or without toppings, as a side dish or mixed into combination dishes—fruits and vegetables are versatile foods. It's just as easy to serve them in heart-healthy ways as it is to serve them loaded with fat and cholesterol. Here's how.

Produce Prep

❑ Save preparation time by using prechopped frozen onions and bell peppers in soup, chili, and casserole recipes. Because of the moisture in them, you can even sauté these time-saving veggies without margarine, oil, or any other liquid.

❑ Use small amounts of low-sodium broth or vegetable oil spray instead of oil to sauté garlic and fresh onions, peppers, mushrooms.

❑ When cooking turnip greens or other greens, you don't need to add pork for flavor. Try a splash of flavored vinegar instead.

❑ Cook vegetables just long enough to make them tender-crisp. Overcooked vegetables lose both flavor and important nutrients.

❑ Stock up on microwaveable containers. This makes it easier to store, cook, and reheat vegetables. When you have extra time, cut up a variety of vegetables, put them in separate containers, and refrigerate. For a meal or snack, just pull out a container, pop the lid slightly, and zap the veggies in the microwave for a few minutes.

❑ Mix chopped fresh or canned fruits (such as apricots, peaches, pineapples, or mangoes) with chopped tomatoes, chopped red onion, and minced garlic for a sassy salsa to accompany chicken or fish.

Who Cooks from Scratch Anymore?

You, for starters. Relax—today, "scratch" cooking
means opening a can, package, or box. For
instance, try a frozen stir-fry kit. Most of these combinations contain vegetables, a soy sauce seasoning, and rice. You just add chicken or low-fat cuts of
pork or beef. It's an easy way to stir up a quick dinner, usually in less than 30 minutes. If you're watching your sodium intake, be aware that the seasoning
packets are often high in sodium. If that's the case,
just discard the packet and use a little low-sodium
soy sauce instead.

Microwave Magic

◆ Use a microwaveable dish that
  can go straight from the oven
  to the table. Doing that will
  save on cleanup time.

◆ Make sure all the food pieces are
  about the same size.

◆ Consult your microwave instruction book or a microwave
  cookbook for guidelines on amounts of water, if any, to use
  in cooking fresh or frozen vegetables.

◆ Cover the dish loosely so that steam can escape.

◆ Unless you're cooking an extra-large amount, you can probably microwave your vegetables on high for 2–13 minutes.
  Experiment with different times or consult charts in
  microwave cookbooks to help you figure out how long to
  cook the veggies.

◆ Let the vegetables stand for a few minutes after microwav-
  ing. That lets them finish cooking and cool slightly.

🅗erb Hint

Because dried herbs are concentrated, it takes less of them than of fresh herbs. As a rule of thumb, 1/4 to 1/3 teaspoon of dried herbs equals 1 teaspoon of fresh. But let your tastebuds be your guide and experiment.

Dress Up Your Vegetables with Herbs and Spices

Try	With
Allspice	Corn, peas, red cabbage, tomatoes, winter squash
Anise	Beets, carrots
Basil	Eggplant, green beans, tomatoes, zucchini
Caraway seeds	Beans, brussels sprouts, cabbage
Chili powder	Cauliflower, corn, peas
Cinnamon	Carrots, sweet potatoes, winter squash
Dill	Carrots, cucumbers, green beans, potatoes
Garlic	Asparagus, cucumbers, greens, spinach, tomatoes
Mint	Beans, carrots, peas
Nutmeg	Carrots, green beans, sweet potatoes, winter squash
Oregano	Eggplant, green beans, mushrooms, spinach, tomatoes, zucchini
Rosemary	Asparagus, cauliflower, corn, mushrooms, peas

BASIL

DILL

ROSEMARY

(continued on next page}

Try	With
Sage	Carrots, peas, tomatoes
Savory	Beans, beets, peas, tomatoes, winter squash
Thyme	Eggplant, green beans, mushrooms, tomatoes, zucchini

SAGE

THYME

Cool and Groovy—The Joys of Frozen Fruit

Experience the taste treat of frozen fruit snacks. After following the preparation tips below, store the fruit in plastic freezer bags with tight-fitting seals. Thaw the fruit slightly before eating it.

◆ Bananas—Peel, then slice into bite-size pieces.

◆ Grapes—Wash and drain thoroughly.

◆ Strawberries—Wash, drain, and cut into bite-size pieces.

Time-Savers

◆ When preparing the pasta for macaroni and (reduced-fat) cheese, add chopped or sliced fresh or frozen vegetables during the last three minutes of boiling. Drain the veggies and macaroni, then complete the recipe as instructed.

*n*icer Rice

Toss a handful or two of raisins into your rice during the last five minutes of cooking. The fruit will add a sweet zing and extra fiber.

◆ Make an extra-large batch of baked vegetables. Preheat your oven to 350° F, then spray a pan with vegetable oil spray. Cut up different veggies, add your favorite nonfat or low-fat seasonings, and bake until tender. Serve the veggies as a side dish one night and use them as the base for a soup, casserole, or stew later in the week. (Hint: Because dense vegetables, such as potatoes, carrots, and parsnips, take longer to cook, cut them into smaller pieces before cooking. Cut softer vegetables, such as zucchini, celery, and mushrooms, into slightly larger pieces.)

♡ Skim Milk and Low-Fat Dairy Products

Whole milk and whole-milk products are high in fat, saturated fat, and cholesterol. Here are some tips to help you keep dairy-related fat and cholesterol under control.

Dairy Gets a Workout

❑ Substitute skim or 1% milk for whole milk in recipes.

❑ Try evaporated skim milk in recipes that call for light cream or half-and-half. It has a thick consistency because evaporation has removed some of the water in the skim milk.

❑ Cut the fat in your casseroles and combination dishes (such as pizza or lasagna) by reducing the amount of cheese. (Some dishes are even great with half the cheese.)

❑ Substitute nonfat or low-fat yogurt for sour cream in dips or on baked potatoes. Or try the new non-fat and low-fat sour cream products.

Cheese Meltdown

Whole-fat cheeses melt more easily than nonfat and low-fat cheeses. Here are some tips to help you compensate.

◆ Mix equal amounts of low-fat or nonfat cheese and regular cheese. The combination will melt, and it will add much less fat and cholesterol than you'd get from using regular cheese by itself.

◆ Add a little water to shredded nonfat cheese. Squeeze 2 to 3 tablespoons of water into 2 cups of shredded cheese. Then sprinkle the cheese on the food and heat.

♡ *Lean Meat, Poultry, Seafood, and Eggs*

Don't spoil your efforts to eat a low-fat diet by loading lean cuts of meat and poultry with lots of fat in the cooking process.

Slimmed-Down Entrées

❑ Remove the skin from poultry and trim all excess fat from meats and poultry *before* cooking. It will cut the amount of fat and saturated fat in half!

❑ After cooking ground meat or ground poultry, drain all the fat. Then put the meat or chicken in a colander and rinse under hot running water.

❑ Leave the bone in when cooking meat and poultry, if possible. It helps retain some of the moisture in lean cuts.

❑ Try grilling and broiling. They're great because they let fat drip away during cooking. First, marinate poultry or tenderized meat to add flavor. You can get even more flavor by basting with a nonfat or low-fat marinade while cooking.

❑ Well-done meat contains less fat than rare meat because the more-cooked meat has been heated enough to melt some of the fat. So, cook your meats until they are medium to well-done. Just make sure to choose a cooking method that allows the fat to drip away.

❑ Filet mignon is a lean beef cut, but many supermarkets and restaurants wrap it in bacon. Do your heart a favor and take the bacon off before cooking the meat.

❑ Use two egg whites for every whole egg in recipes, or use egg substitute.

Gravy Train

Skim the fat off meat and poultry drippings for broths and gravies. Here are a few techniques to help get the fat out of the gravy.

◆ Chill the drippings, which lets the fat rise to the top. Then spoon off the congealed fat.

◆ Use a gravy separator, which looks like a measuring cup with the pouring spout at the bottom. Pour the drippings into the separator, wait 10 to 15 minutes for the fat to rise to the top, and then pour the broth from the bottom, stopping when the fat reaches the spout.

◆ Make your own gravy separator. Place an airtight 1-quart plastic freezer bag in a small bowl. Pour in the cooled drippings, zip the bag closed, and let the drippings sit for 10 to 15 minutes. Holding the bag over the bowl, snip a small hole in one of the bag's bottom corners. Stop the flow after the broth has run out. Discard the bag with the fat.

Love Me Tender

Lean meat has less fat, saturated fat, and cholesterol than fattier meat has. However, it's less tender than fattier cuts if you cook it the same way you cook a fatty steak. Here are some ways to make even the leanest meat tender.

◆ Pound it evenly with a meat mallet.

◆ Marinate it. An acidic mixture helps break down the fibers. Marinades can add a nice change of flavor, too. Try

   • nonfat or low-fat salad dressings
   • flavorful vinegars
   • wine
   • picante sauce or salsa
   • citrus fruits, such as lemons, limes, and oranges

Remember, boil the marinade before using it to baste the meat during cooking. That will kill any bacteria from the raw meat.

◆ Slice it against the grain.

Escape from Takeout Prison

Does your busy schedule hold you hostage to drive-through burger pickup and fried chicken takeout? If so, get smart. Use the weekends to get ahead with meal preparation. Here's a weekend plan for a family of four:

On Saturday:

◆ Buy

- 12 skinless chicken breast halves
- Nonfat French dressing
- Nonfat Italian dressing
- Nonfat honey Dijon dressing

On Sunday:

◆ Marinate 4 pieces in each of the dressings for at least four hours.

◆ Bake or broil all 12 pieces.

◆ Serve 4 pieces for dinner.

◆ Refrigerate the remaining 8 pieces for reheating later in the week.

Easy Steamed Shrimp

Buy fresh shrimp at the supermarket seafood counter and have it steamed while you shop. Keep the shrimp chilled at home for up to two days, then enjoy an easy, quick entrée.

Dollar-Stretching Strategy

You can get more burgers, sloppy Joes, or tacos—and less fat—for your money by stretching your ground beef or turkey. Add small amounts of starchy fillers, such as dry quick-cooking oatmeal, cooked rice, mashed potatoes, finely chopped or shredded vegetables, or bread crumbs.

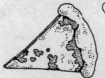

♡ Now and Then— Foods from the Tip of the Pyramid

Fat-cutting food preparation ideas abound for this category. We'll cover them with cooking tips and ideas for how to deal with a major snack attack.

Baker's Rack

❑ Cut the saturated fat in your baking by using liquid oil rather than solid vegetable shortening or butter.

❑ Look for pastry recipes that use vegetable oil instead of butter or shortening.

❑ Trim the fat by replacing part of the shortening in a recipe with applesauce or apple butter. This works especially well in cookie recipes. Try using plain nonfat or low-fat yogurt instead of oil in brownie mixes.

Snack Attack Know-How

❏ One ounce of potato chips (about 15 chips) has about 150 calories and 10 grams of fat. But can you stop at 15 chips? Instead, try

◆ Reduced-fat varieties that have about 140 calories and 6.7 grams of fat

◆ Baked varieties that have about 110 calories and 1.5 grams of fat

◆ Fat-free potato chips that have about 110 calories and less than 1 gram of fat.

Good-bye, Mr. Chips

❏ If you think that potato chips are your only snack chip option, think again. Instead, try

◆ Bagel chips—Lay any flavor of bagel flat on a cutting board. Refrigerated or day-old bagels work best. Carefully make vertical cuts through the bagel. Each piece should be a small circle or oval that is ⅛- to ¼-inch thick. Place the slices on an ungreased baking sheet. Bake at 350° F for 10 to 12 minutes, or until crisp and light brown.

Triple Dip

Make your favorite dip using nonfat or re-duced-fat sour cream or plain yogurt. Blend nonfat or low-fat cottage cheese in the food processor for a third yummy option.

- ◆ Corn tortilla chips—Cut corn tortillas into six wedges each. Place the wedges on an ungreased baking sheet. Bake at 400° F for 10 to 11 minutes, or until crisp. Bring on the salsa!

- ◆ Pita chips—Split pita pockets in half lengthwise and then cut into wedges. Toast the wedges at 325° F for 8 minutes, or until crisp.

Popcorn Potential

Popcorn can be a terrific snack depending on how you pop it.

Regular microwave (2 cups)	**3–7 g of fat**
Popped in oil (2 cups)	**3–4 g of fat**
Light microwave (2 cups)	**1–2 g of fat**
Air popped (2 cups)	**Less than 1 g of fat**

Want Some Popcorn with Your Fat?

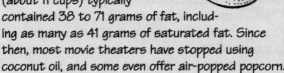

Before May 1994, most movie theaters popped their popcorn in coconut oil, a highly saturated fat. A medium tub of movie theater popcorn (about 11 cups) typically contained 38 to 71 grams of fat, including as many as 41 grams of saturated fat. Since then, most movie theaters have stopped using coconut oil, and some even offer air-popped popcorn.

*S*mile and Say "Parmesan"

Try lightly seasoning your air-popped popcorn with herbs or a sprinkle of Parmesan cheese.

Eating Out—Eating Healthy

Making healthful choices at restaurants is becoming easier. Because of consumer demand, lots of restaurants now offer more-healthful options. Restaurants want their food to taste good, and many are finding ways to make that happen without sending the fat content off the charts. Here are some ideas to help you navigate your way through the menu.

Ordering à la Heart

❑ Be assertive and politely ask for what you want. Request margarine instead of butter, vegetables without butter, and dry toast.

❑ Ask that gravies, sauces, and salad dressings be served on the side. Then you can control how much you eat.

❑ Ask how food is prepared. Many restaurants are willing to accommodate special requests for preparing food. For example, if the menu lists fried fish, see if yours can be broiled or baked instead. You can also ask for the fat to be trimmed from meats and for the skin to be removed from poultry before cooking.

❑ Mexican restaurants are popular these days, but your server invariably greets you with a bottom-less basket of tortilla chips. So the next time you're hankering for south-of-the-border cuisine, ask for a few warm corn tortillas instead to dip in the salsa—and save big on fat grams.

❑ Investigate the descriptions of each dish on the menu. If you're sharp, you'll notice unmistakable clues to high-fat and low-fat foods (see the chart below for some sleuthing tips).

Be a Menu Detective

High-Fat Clues	Low-Fat Clues
Au gratin; in cheese sauce; Parmesan	Au jus; in its own juices
Buttered; buttery	Baked
Breaded and fried	Broiled, with lemon
Casserole	juice or wine
Creamed; creamy; in cream sauce	Fresh; garden fresh
Fried; French fried; deep fried;	Grilled
batter fried; pan fried; crispy	Lean
Gravy; pan gravy	Poached
Hash	Roasted
Hollandaise	Steamed
Pastry	
Pot pie	
Rich	
Sautéed	
Scalloped; escalloped	

How to "Cheat"

Bet that got your attention! You'd better sit down, because this chapter may shock you. After learning lots of strategies for getting the fat out of your diet, now you're going to learn how to "cheat"—and still keep a healthful fat level. Can't be done? Oh, yes it can!

Healthful eating is knowing what to eat, knowing how much to eat, and then following through *consistently*. That means at least 80% of the time. But reality delivers special occasions, circumstances when low-fat food isn't available, and cravings for a food that's not on your list of low-fat favorites. In this chapter, you'll find out how to deal with these situations. You'll also learn how to make nutrition trade-offs. With a little know-how, you can cheat in a way that won't do permanent damage to your overall fat-lowering plan. Your cheatin' heart won't tell on you.

♡ Breads, Cereals, Pasta, and Starchy Vegetables

As much as you want to cut down on fat, remember that *your goal is not a fat-free diet*. That's unrealistic and 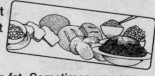 undesirable. You need *some* fat. Sometimes you can mix a high-fat food with a low-fat food to create a healthful and delicious combination.

Mixed Blessings

❑ Mix 3 tablespoons of nonfat yogurt and 1 table-spoon of pimiento cheese. Let this melt into a piping hot spud. It's luscious but low in fat!

❑ Mix higher-fat cereals, such as granola, with cere-als lower in fat. You'll capture different tastes and textures yet keep your fat intake low.

❑ Compensate for a high-fat muf-fin or biscuit by making the rest of your meal low fat.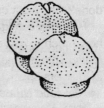

❑ Think of a favorite food that you tend to limit because it's high in fat. Figure out ways to adjust, mix, or modify it.

❑ Consider ways to reduce calories, particularly in the starch group. One idea is to mix spaghetti squash with angel hair pasta. This cuts the calo-ries and adds texture and different nutrients to a favorite Italian dish.

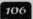

♡ *Vegetables and Fruits*

Even though it's Week 5, you may still be having trouble eating enough fruits and vegetables. Here are some simple solutions.

Veggie Loading

❑ Case your grocer's freezer for individual servings of frozen veggies. These are super to throw in your lunch bag and microwave at work.

❑ Can't give up smothering your vegetables with cheese sauce? Then cut the fat and sodium in half by mixing one package of frozen vegetables with cheese sauce and a second package of vegetables without sauce.

❑ Order extra side dishes of steamed vegetables when eating out. Perk up the flavor with a squirt of fresh lemon or lime.

Tantalizing Topping Tips

Steamed veggies too bland? Use lemon or jazz them up with one of these great toppings.

◆ *Parmesan cheese.* Sprinkle a small amount on hot vegetables. The pungent flavor makes a little go a long way. And try grated instead of shredded—it will go even farther.

◆ *Light processed cheese.* Cut into small cubes and melt them in your microwave. Pour over hot vegetables.

◆ *Balsamic vinegar.* A mild but flavorful vinegar, it's great for salads and vegetables alike.

◆ *Garlic.* Sauté 2 cloves of minced garlic in 1 teaspoon of
   olive oil. Stir into hot vegetables.

Eat Your Spinach!

Do your kids boycott vegetables? Try these tactics.

◆ Get your kids involved in preparing
   vegetables and salads. If you have
   a garden, let the children discover
   how seeds become food. Let
   them pick their own food from the
   garden, rinse it, and eat it right
   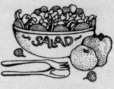
   away. There's no need to wait until dinner for a healthful
   serving of fresh vegetables.

◆ Keep vegetables tender-crisp. Don't overcook!

◆ Let kids eat vegetables as finger foods they can dip in nonfat or low-fat dressings.

◆ Sneak vegetables into other foods, such as casseroles,
   meat sauce, and even muffins.

*B*erry Good!

Top your frozen yogurt or ice milk with berries
or other fruits instead of nuts or candy.

♡ *Skim Milk and Low-Fat Dairy Products*

Though nonfat and low-fat dairy delights abound,
sometimes you may want the richer version. Give in

to your urge and splurge *occasionally*, while keeping the following tips in mind.

We All Scream for Ice Cream

❑ If you're going to eat regular or premium ice cream every once in a while, measure a half-cup into a small bowl. The size of the bowl will make your serving look larger. A delicious optical illusion!

❑ Buy only small containers of ice cream. Then there won't be a lot of extra fat and cholesterol waiting around to be eaten.

❑ Remember that ice cream isn't your only option. Take a look at the nonfat and low-fat frozen dessert alternatives listed below.

Truly Cool Frozen Desserts

	Total Fat (g)	Saturated Fat (g)	Cholesterol (mg)	Calories
Frozen yogurt, low-fat (½ cup)	4.0	2.5	2	114
Frozen yogurt, nonfat (½ cup)	0.0	0.0	0.0	110
Ice milk (½ cup)	2.8	1.7	9	92
Sherbet (½ cup)	1.7	1.0	4	97
Sorbet (½ cup)	0.0	0.0	0.0	120

How to Strike Oil

So you couldn't convince your friends to order a
pizza with less cheese? Before you dive in, grab a
few paper napkins and sop up the oil that's sitting on
the melted cheese. You could save yourself several
grams of fat per slice.

♡ *Lean Meat,*
  Poultry, Seafood,
  and Eggs

Foods in this group provide as much as half the fat
in the average American diet. It's still possible to
enjoy a Prime or Choice cut of meat from time to
time, *if* you follow these guidelines.

Grade "A" Ideas

❑ If you eat a higher-fat entrée, eat lower-fat foods
   with it. Also try to eat lower-fat meals for the rest
   of the day.

❑ Save fattier cuts of meat and foods such as fried
   chicken for special occasions—your anniversary,
   your birthday, or a promotion. Eating high-fat
   entrées this infrequently is not likely to harm you.
   But be careful not to use everyone else's anniver-
   saries and birthdays as excuses to indulge!

❑ If you can't avoid having a fatty cut of meat or a
   piece of fried fish (you're at your in-laws' house,

for example), try to eat a smaller serving than you normally would.

☐ You may be getting extra fat and cholesterol from oversized hamburger patties. But sometimes you really want a hamburger. Solution? Simple! Watch your portion size. Buy exactly one pound of lean ground beef and divide it evenly into four patties. That's the maximum size you should shoot for.

Food in the Fast Lane

It's going to be a fast-food night. No way to get around it. So what are your best chicken choices? Look at the chart on page 111 for some comparisons.

ℋefty Heifers

People aren't the only ones watching their figures. So are cattle and hogs. New feeding and breeding practices have created beef cattle and hogs that are leaner than ever before. For example, on average, pork today is 31% leaner than it was 10 years ago.

♡ *Now and Then—Foods from the Tip of the Pyramid*

While we're focusing on trade-offs and coping techniques for following a low-fat eating plan, what food

Fast-Food Chicken Pickin's

	Total Fat (g)	Saturated Fat (g)	Cholesterol (mg)	Calories
Rotisserie (baked) chicken (breast and drumstick) without skin	7.1	2.2	151	289
Rotisserie (baked) chicken (breast and drumstick) with skin	17.2	4.9	173	405
Grilled chicken filet sandwich	18.0	3.0	53	379
Fried chicken filet sandwich	40.0	8.0	82	685
Chicken nuggets (1 order, 6 pieces)	13.0	3.0	46	236
Fried chicken, regular (breast and drumstick)	23.8	6.0	160	429
Fried chicken, extra crispy (breast and drumstick)	33.6	8.2	185	546

group is more relevant than this? Here are some
ways to make small amounts of the foods from this
group part of your low-fat eating plan.

𝑛 uts

If you love nuts, you'll go nuts when you learn how much fat they contain. Example? Two tablespoons of peanut butter contain 16 grams of fat and 188 calories.

Snacking Smart

❑ Since most people tend to snack spontaneously, anticipate the times and places most likely to bring on your snack attacks. Then plan ahead to have nonfat or low-fat snacks on hand.

❑ If you're in a situation where healthful snacking is impossible, choose your food carefully the rest of the day to adjust for the extra fat, calories, and sodium in your snacks.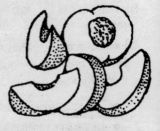

❑ During a snack attack, ask yourself, "Is this food worth the calories and fat?" It might be, if your overall diet is very low in fat and/or a particular food is absolutely your favorite. On the other hand, the indulgence may not be worth the consequences. All things considered, you may be just as satisfied with a lower-fat option.

❑ If you love a particular food yet feel you can't afford its extra fat and calories, consider taking only a bite or two. The challenge here is to keep the amount to one or two bites, not three, four, or the whole serving.

The Nuts and Bolts of Nuts and Fat

❑ Limit the amount of nuts and seeds you add to your salad. Just 1 ounce of sunflower seeds contains 16 grams of fat. If you love 'em, use just a sprinkle. Chop nuts into very small pieces to make a little go a longer way.

❑ Buy pretzels and low-fat whole-wheat crackers instead of peanuts to munch on for a snack. Remember: What you put in your pantry will end up in your mouth.

❑ If you're a true peanut butter lover, there's really nuttin' to worry about. Just

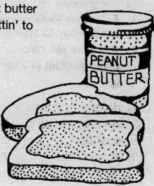

◆ Spread it thinner.

◆ Try the light varieties.

◆ Try the natural type that separates, and pour off some of the oil.

◆ Use a filler. Example: Add cooked carrots to the peanut butter. You still get the peanut butter flavor and texture but not as much fat.

Sweet Nothings

These traditional desserts offer few nutrients but plenty of fat and calories.

	Fat (g)	Calories
Premium ice cream (1 cup)	20	300
Fudge cake with icing ($\frac{1}{10}$ of cake)	17	437
Cheesecake ($\frac{1}{6}$ of cake)	16	341
Chocolate candy bar ($1\frac{1}{2}$ oz)	13	238
Gingerbread (1 piece)	13	267
Apple pie ($\frac{1}{6}$ of pie)	11	250
Danish pastry (1 piece)	9	161
Brownie (2" x $2\frac{1}{2}$")	8	167
Chocolate chip cookies (2)	5	92

♡ *Eating Out—Eating Healthy*

Few things are as tempting as eating at your favorite restaurant, particularly on special occasions. Use the following pointers to help make dining out a heart-healthy success.

À la Heart

❏ If you're dining out for a special occasion, save your fat grams by eating a light breakfast and lunch. Then you can splurge a bit at dinner.

❑ Many special occasion dinners include a cocktail, an appetizer, and a dessert. Decide ahead of time to have only one of the three. You can still have a fabulous dining-out experience.

Dessert Tray

Many people have the philosophy, "Life is short. Eat dessert first." If you're among them, there's no reason to deprive yourself. The following sweet-eating strategies can help your heart as well as please your palate.

Sweet Inspirations

❑ Share a dessert. Sometimes restaurant portions of desserts are enormous. It can be a lot of fun to order one dessert for two, three, or even four people. To satisfy a sweet tooth, often a little dab will do ya!

❑ Choose a fruit-based dessert.

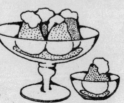

❑ Choose a light dessert, such as angel food cake and berries or frozen yogurt.

Drink and Grow Fat

Though alcohol contains no fat, it's loaded with empty calories. If you drink alcohol while trying to lose weight, you may end up crying in your beer. The smartest plan is to avoid or limit alcoholic drinks.

Take a look at the chart below to see just how many calories are in some drinks.

Popular Drinks

	Calories
Alcohol-free beer (12 oz)	65
Beer, regular (12 oz)	150
Beer, light (12 oz)	100
Bloody Mary (5 oz)	125
Champagne (4 oz)	85
Gin and tonic (8 oz)	155
Margarita (8 oz)	300
Martini (3½ oz)	140
Wine (3½ oz)	85

Tricks of the Trade

You're in the homestretch! All you need is a few final tips for continuing your fat- and cholesterol-cutting game plan.

This week, you'll learn about meatless meals as a way to decrease fat and increase carbohydrates. You'll also get more heart-healthy fruit and vegetable strategies. And you'll find tips on taming the chocolate monster and eating at fast-food restaurants. All are great ideas to help you keep cutting fat and cholesterol for life!

♡ Breads, Cereals, Pasta, and Starchy Vegetables

Don't know beans about beans? Some people think that beans are fattening, but that's not true. Actually, a half-cup of beans contains only about 100 to 150 calories and just a trace of fat. Beans are much

lower in calories than meat is, and they provide nearly as much protein. If you're like most other
Americans, you don't eat nearly enough fiber.
Fortunately, beans are also a great source of fiber.
Fiber can help lower blood cholesterol when eaten
as part of a diet that is low in saturated fat. Finally,
beans are amazingly inexpensive.

Bean Bag

❑ Try some beans or peas you haven't tried before.

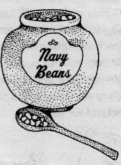

- ◆ Black beans (turtle beans)
- ◆ Black-eyed peas
- ◆ Garbanzo beans (chick-peas)
- ◆ Great Northern beans (Northern white beans)
- ◆ Kidney beans
- ◆ Lentils
- ◆ Lima beans
- ◆ Mung beans, sprouted
- ◆ Navy beans
- ◆ Pinto beans
- ◆ Soybeans
- ◆ Split peas

❑ Combine beans or peas with rice or another grain
for complete-protein meatless meals.

Spilling the Beans about Beans

◆ Dried beans need to be well rinsed before cooking. The
package may contain small pebbles, bits of soil, or other
debris.

◆ Most dried beans need to soak for at least a couple of hours before cooking. If you're in a time crunch, you can boil the beans for two to three minutes and then soak them for about an hour before cooking.

◆ Canned beans are convenient. Drain and rinse them in a colander to reduce the sodium content.

◆ A common complaint with beans is that they can produce gas. To reduce gas significantly, discard the water after soaking the beans. Then cook the beans in a large quantity of water and discard the cooking water as well.

♡ Vegetables and Fruits

Over the six weeks of this program, we have offered a host of ideas for adding heart-healthy fruits and vegetables to your eating plan. If you've tried even a third of the suggestions, you're well on your 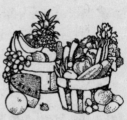 way to a high-fiber, low-fat diet. Here are a few last-minute tips and a challenge to test your fruit and veggie savvy.

Staying Ahead of the Game

❑ Turn your plain old salad into a one-dish meal by adding leftover chicken breast, lean roast beef, or reduced-fat ham; potatoes, pasta, or rice; and lots of veggies or some mandarin oranges, strawberries, or raspberries.

❏ Fire up the grill for . . . vegetables? Why not? Toss them on the grill, with or without being marinated. Firm vegetables, such as sweet potatoes, may need to be precooked slightly.

❏ Does eating pancakes or a waffle without margarine or syrup sound like medieval torture? Try pureed fruits, such as bananas and strawberries, as a topping instead. It's a great way to have your cakes and eat your fruit, too.

❏ Fruits and vegetables are virtually fat free, so fill up on them. If you're getting tired of the same old apples, bananas, oranges, and broccoli:

- ◆ Let your tastebuds dance a tango with a mango;
- ◆ "Pear up" with a Bartlett pear;
- ◆ Let passion fruit bring out the best in you;
- ◆ Kiss a kiwifruit; or
- ◆ Dive into a bowl of endive.

Take the Fruit and Veggie Challenge

Try your hand at thinking of heart-healthy ways to add more fruits and vegetables to your diet. (Turn to page 123 for hints.)

◆ Three ways to enjoy vegetables *before* lunch:

_____

_____

_____

_____

◆ Three ways to include vegetables and fruits in party menus:

_____

_____

_____

◆ Three ways to get fruits and vegetables at a fast-food
restaurant or convenience store:

_____

_____

_____

◆ Three ways to order vegetables or salad when eating at a
sit-down, white-tablecloth restaurant:

_____

_____

_____

◆ Five strategies for making vegetables more convenient:

_____

_____

_____

_____

_____

◆ Four tasty mixtures of dairy products and fruit:

_____

_____

_____

_____

◆ Three ways to "sneak" a serving of vegetables into other foods:

_____

_____

_____

◆ Three creative ways to get your kids to eat their veggies:

_____

_____

_____

◆ Three ways to get fruits and vegetables when traveling:

_____

_____

_____

◆ Five toppings to make vegetables more appealing and tastier:

_____

_____

_____

_____

_____

Answers to the Fruit and Veggie Challenge

By no means are these the only answers to this heart-healthy challenge. But they may give you new ideas.

Three ways to enjoy vegetables *before* lunch:

1. Glass of tomato or vegetable juice.

2. Carrot sticks and nonfat or low-fat dip.

3. Celery sticks stuffed with nonfat or low-fat cream cheese.

Three ways to include vegetables and fruits in holiday party menus:

1. Vegetable tray with nonfat or low-fat dip.

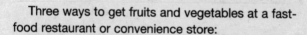

2. Low-fat pumpkin pie (pumpkin is a vegetable and is packed with vitamin A!).

3. Extra fruit added to molded salads.

Three ways to get fruits and vegetables at a fast-food restaurant or convenience store:

1. Fresh whole fruit (apples, oranges, bananas).

2. Premade salads with nonfat or low-fat dressing.

3. Fruit or vegetable juice.

Three ways to order vegetables or a salad when eating at a sit-down, white-tablecloth restaurant:

1. "Dressing on the side, please."

2. "Steamed vegetables without butter or oil, please."

3. "Extra serving of vegetables, please, without added oils or sauces."

Five strategies for making vegetables more convenient:

1. Buy precut vegetables or packaged salads.

2. Cut vegetables and package them in single-serving bags for lunches.

3. Use frozen or canned vegetables without added salt or fat.

4. Make a big pot of vegetable-rich soup, and enjoy it for several quick meals during the week.

5. Drink your veggies! Keep cans of vegetable juice handy for a quick dose of total nutrition.

Four tasty mixtures of dairy products and fruit:

1. Apple slices and nonfat or low-fat Cheddar cheese.

2. Nonfat or low-fat cottage cheese and canned peaches or fresh cantaloupe.

3. Fruit and yogurt smoothie.

4. Nonfat or low-fat yogurt topped with fresh fruit.

Three ways to "sneak" a serving of vegetables into other foods:

1. Grated carrots in meat loaf.

2. Chopped veggies (such as broccoli, cauliflower, and green peppers) in spaghetti or taco sauces.

3. Tomatoes, mushrooms, sprouts, green peppers, and dark-green lettuce added to sandwiches or burgers.

Three creative ways to get your kids to eat their veggies:

1. Include small pieces of broccoli, cauliflower, zucchini, and/or other vegetables in soups and casseroles.

2. Make "Ants on a Log." Fill celery sticks with nonfat or low-fat cream cheese and top with raisins ("ants").

3. Serve raw veggies and a favorite nonfat or low-fat dip. Kids love to dip foods.

Three ways to get your fruits and vegetables when traveling:

1. Carry dried fruit with you.

2. Always have juice at breakfast.

3. Make lunchtime "salad time."

Five different toppings to make vegetables more appealing and tastier:

1. Nonfat or low-fat cheese.

2. Small amounts of grated Parmesan cheese.

3. Fat-free or low-fat salad dressings.

4. Garlic powder.

5. Balsamic vinegar.

♡ Skim Milk and Low-Fat Dairy Products

Here are a few final tips to help you with this food group.

Put Dairy on a Diet

❑ By switching from 1% milk to skim milk, you'll save 11,680 calories, 1,606 grams of fat, and 949 grams of saturated fat each year (assuming you drink 2 cups of milk a day)!

❑ Additional flavors of nonfat and low-fat yogurt hit the dairy case every year. Explore the new options. You may find one that you can't live without!

❑ Less is more if you use the sharpest variety of cheese available. You can use a smaller amount but still have lots of cheese flavor.

❑ Thanks to consumer demand, nonfat cream, cottage, and ricotta cheeses are now available. Try them in dips, spreads, cheesecakes, and casseroles.

❑ Try feta cheese. It's a low-fat cheese that crumbles nicely over soups and salads. Also, its pungent flavor means you don't have to use much.

♡ Lean Meat, Poultry, Seafood, and Eggs

At the beginning of this book, we stressed eating lean meat, poultry, and seafood. Then we challenged you to eat smaller portions. Now we want to encourage you to eat meat, poultry, and seafood less often. No, it's not necessary to become a vegetarian. Simply explore meatless options at least a few times a month.

Don't Chicken Out on Meatless Meals

❏ Try to eat at least a couple of meatless meals a month.

❏ Try a meatless meal made up of vegetables with a variety of textures. You might start with grilled portobello mushrooms. Believe it or not, they remind many people of steak and are terrific served on a bun!

❏ Most vegetarian products are low in saturated fat and cholesterol. But not all are low in total fat. Read the label to be sure you choose low-fat meatless products.

Do You Need Meat Every Day to Be Healthy?

No. It's true that beef, poultry, and seafood are good sources of protein, iron, zinc, and other important nutrients. But you can get many of these same nutrients from other foods, such as nonfat and low-fat dairy products, dried beans and peas (kidney, pinto, navy, lentils, etc.), and dark-green leafy vegetables. All these meatless foods are low in fat and cholesterol. So meatless meals can be a highly effective heart-healthy strategy.

Meatless Entrées: Better Than Ever

Try products that imitate the flavor and texture of meat but are totally meatless. Some are made from soybeans, and others are combinations of vegetables flavored and shaped to look like the meaty original. These products may be high in sodium, however. Read the label to see just how much sodium is in each serving. If it's more than you want, look for a lower-sodium alternative or select very low sodium foods for the rest of the day.

We've listed several of these meatless products below. Grocery stores stock many of them in the freezer case. You may have to look for other products in health-food stores.

- ◆ Bacon
- ◆ Breakfast sausage
- ◆ Burgers
- ◆ Burritos
- ◆ Cold cuts
- ◆ Hot dogs
- ◆ Tacos

Down with Fat, Up with Money

Surimi is a protein-packed, low-fat fish product sold as a low-cost alternative to crab legs.

♡ Now and Then—Foods from the Tip of the Pyramid

This section of *6 Weeks to Get Out the Fat* is dedicated to the food of the gods, chocolate. Many people have resolved that this substance, at 9 grams of fat per ounce, will never again pass their lips. Until they are tempted by the next chocolate cheesecake!

Chocolate cravings are a part of life. You just have to know how to handle them.

Stop, in the Name of Love!

❑ Try a 1½-ounce chocolate-covered peppermint patty instead of a 1½-ounce chocolate bar. You'll save about 9 grams of fat and about 100 calories.

❑ Have a chocolate urge? Stop by a convenience store and buy only three bite-size pieces of chocolate candy. That little bit of chocolate will probably satisfy your urge to splurge. And you saved yourself from the fat overload you'd get with a larger candy bar.

❑ Two tablespoons of chocolate syrup contain approximately 73 calories and less than ½ gram of fat. Hot fudge sauce, though, contains 10 grams of fat per quarter-cup. For a low-fat snack, stir the syrup into a glass of skim milk or pour it over nonfat or low-fat frozen yogurt.

❑ Cocoa powder is an excellent substitute for chocolate in baking. Use 3 tablespoons of cocoa powder plus 1 tablespoon of vegetable oil for every ounce of chocolate in a recipe. You'll cut the fat in half.

Chocolate Chips

◆ Chocolate-dipped fruit tastes great, but is it worth the fat grams? A dipped strawberry is coated with about ¼ ounce of chocolate (2.3 grams of fat). Two chocolate-covered cherries contain about 4.5 grams of fat, and 2 tablespoons of chocolate-covered raisins contain about 4.8 grams of fat.

◆ Chocolate-covered pretzels, graham crackers, and malted milk balls have about half the fat of chocolate-covered nuts.

◆ Carob has only one advantage over chocolate. Carob does not contain caffeine. Both a carob bar and a chocolate bar contain about 150 calories and 9 grams of fat per ounce.

♡ *Eating Out—Eating Healthy*

Studies show that the average fast-food meal adds up to about 1,200 calories! But you don't have to give up fast foods completely to eat heart-healthy. Just be selective.

Life in the Fast-Food Lane

❏ Order a small hamburger instead of a specialty burger.

❏ Order roast beef for a leaner choice than most burgers.

❑ Order a grilled chicken or fish sandwich in place of fried chicken or a fried fish sandwich. Calories can more than double with deep-fried choices.

❑ To reduce fat, omit mayonnaise, cheese, bacon, and special sauces from your sandwich. Instead, choose toppings such as mustard, tomatoes, lettuce, pickles, and onions.

❑ Select a baked potato instead of French fries. Top it with cottage cheese, picante sauce, 2 tablespoons of grated cheese or sour cream, or chili.

❑ Order a salad or create a salad at the salad bar. Eat lots of deep-green lettuce or spinach, raw vegetables, and beans. Limit cheese, fried noodles, bacon bits, nuts, and seeds. Use vinegar and a small amount of oil, or choose a nonfat or low-fat dressing.

❑ Order pizza with vegetable toppings, such as peppers, mushrooms, or onions, instead of extra cheese, pepperoni, or sausage. Eat two to three pieces and have a salad.

❑ Avoid high-calorie beverages. Instead of regular soft drinks and milk shakes, order skim or 1% milk, vegetable or fruit juice, tea, or water.

❑ Order fat-free bakery products, such as a fat-free apple muffin. Remember to watch your calories. Some fat-free products contain even more calories than the higher-fat version.

❑ Try nonfat or low-fat frozen yogurt or a small nonfat or low-fat milk shake for dessert.

Small Changes, Big Difference

	Typical Order	Modified Order
Sandwich	Specialty burger	Regular hamburger
Side order	Large French fries	½ small order French fries
Beverage	12-oz soft drink	Unsweetened iced tea
Dessert	Milk shake	Low-fat frozen yogurt cone
Total Fat	64 g	15.5 g
Saturated Fat	25.2 g	16.1 g
Cholesterol	150 mg	44.5 mg
Calories	1,436	475

Putting It All Together

Now that you've worked through this book, we hope you've found many good ideas for cutting fat and cholesterol and have put them to work for you. In fact, you may have already seen positive health changes, such as much-needed weight loss or a reduction in your blood pressure or blood cholesterol level. Take a look at "Planning for Change" on page 33. Did you list your strategies and rewards? Did you accomplish the goals you set? If so, go ahead—reward yourself. You deserve it!

Yes, you're certainly in the homestretch, but don't shelve this book just yet! First, you'll want to make sure that you can maintain your new low-fat, low-cholesterol eating habits for life. How? Start by keeping this book handy so that you can easily add a trick or two to your repertoire. For example, you probably couldn't try *all* the tips in *all* the food groups each week. We even strongly advised you to focus on only a few tips at a time. Not to worry! In the coming weeks and months, pick up this book and find sections you may have bypassed the first time around. Or look for sections where you made only a few check marks. Try a couple of new fat-busting tips from one of the sections. Practice those tips until they, too, become habits. Eventually, you'll be an expert in getting out the fat.

♡ How to Make Your Changes Last a Lifetime

Now that you have adopted some new healthful habits, you want to avoid slipping back into old habits over time. Here are some ideas to maintain your new, heart-healthy practices.

Take small steps.   Don't bite off more than you can chew. It's a lot easier when you give yourself time to "digest" new tactics and habits.

Include friends and family.   It's no fun (and less successful) to "fly solo." When changing your way of eating, enlist friends and family. After all, most meals are social events as well as times to refuel your body. Don't underestimate the power of mutual support.

Plan ahead to avoid slips.   Changing your eating habits is sometimes a "two steps forward, one step backward" process. Try to anticipate those situations that can trip you up. And if you do slip, find out what triggered the lapse and learn from your experience.

Give yourself pats on the back. It feels good to achieve a heart-healthy eating goal. So reward yourself for a job well done. This makes it more fun to try new challenges!

Assess your progress. Nothing motivates like success. Track your eating habits and health status from time to time. For example:

◆ Retake the "Fat IQ" quiz beginning on page 10. See how your score differs from your starting score. Chances are it's higher. Progress: It makes you feel good and helps keep you motivated.

◆ Have your blood cholesterol level checked periodically. Reducing fat, especially saturated fat, and cholesterol is a major strategy for lowering blood cholesterol levels. If you've made heart-healthy dietary changes, you probably will see a drop in your blood cholesterol level. Lower blood cholesterol means less risk of heart disease. What better reward can you have for your fat-fighting efforts?

Fortunately, resources abound that can help you maintain your heart-healthy eating habits and even pick up a few new ideas. For example, take a look at our heart-healthy cookbooks:

◆ *The American Heart Association Cookbook, Fifth Edition*
◆ *The American Heart Association Low-Fat, Low-Cholesterol Cookbook*

- *The American Heart Association Low-Salt Cookbook*
- *The American Heart Association Kids' Cookbook*
- *The American Heart Association Quick and Easy Cookbook*

Contact the American Heart Association at 1-800-AHA-USA1 (1-800-242-8721) or online at http://www.amhrt.org for more information about these and other low-fat, low-cholesterol resources.

Bon Appétit!

In a few short weeks you've done a lot to improve your diet—and your health. Remember that good nutrition is knowing what to eat and how much to eat. Then put that knowledge to work for you consistently, at least 80% of the time. Now you know what thousands of other people know. Low-fat, low-cholesterol eating can be delicious—and can help your heart at the same time. *Bon appétit!*

APPENDIX

Where to Reach Us

For information about the American Heart Association, call 1-800-AHA-USA1 (1-800-242-8721) or contact us online at http!//www.amhrt.org

INDEX

A

Alcohol, 115–16

B

Balanced diet, 27, 28, 30, 72-85

Beans, 117–19. *See also* Starchy vegetables

Beef. *See* Meat

Breads
  calories in, 37, 38
  cheating with, 105
  choosing, 35–38
  and eating out, 71
  fat in, 37, 38
  using crumbs as fillers, 99
  labels for, 36
  servings of, 28, 29, 57–59
  spreads for, 87
  variety with, 72–74

Butter. *See* Margarine and butter

C

Calcium, 64–66

Calories, 34, 56, 85, 130. *See also type of food*

Cereals
  cheating with, 105
  choosing, 35–37
  servings of, 28, 29, 57–59
  as snacks, 83
  variety with, 73–74, 79

Cheese, 42, 44, 45, 65, 87–88, 94, 95, 106, 109, 126. *See also* Dairy products

Chocolate, 129–30

Cookbooks, AHA, 135–36

D

Dairy products
  and calcium, 64, 65–66
  cheating with, 107–9
  choosing, 41–45

139